Indispensable
Guides to
Clinical
Practice

Second edition

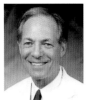

Alan Menter MD
Chief, Department of Dermatology
Baylor Medical Center, Dallas and
Clinical Professor, University of Texas
Southwestern Medical School, Dallas, USA

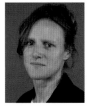

Catherine Smith MD FRCP
Senior Lecturer and Consultant Dermatologist
St John's Institute of Dermatology
St Thomas' Hospital, London, UK

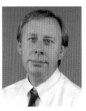

Jonathan Barker MD FRCP FRCPath
Professor of Clinical Dermatology and
Head of Division of Skin Sciences
St John's Institute of Dermatology
St Thomas' Hospital, London, UK

This book is as balanced and as practical as we can make it. Ideas for improvements are always welcome: feedback@fastfacts.com

HEALTH PRESS
Oxford

D1584874

Fast Facts – Psoriasis
First published April 2002
Second edition October 2004

Book orders can be placed by telephone or via the website.
For regional distributors or to order via the website, please go to:
www.fastfacts.com
For telephone orders, please call 01752 202301 (UK), +44 1752 202301 (Europe) or
800 538 1287 (North America, toll free).

Alan Menter acknowledges the assistance of Dr Chris Cather in the review of
chapters 2, 3, 6 and 7.

A CIP catalogue record for this title is available from the British Library.

ISBN 1-903734-56-8

Menter, A (Alan)
Fast Facts – Psoriasis/
Alan Menter, Catherine Smith, Jonathan Barker

Illustrated by Dee McLean, London, UK.
Typesetting and page layout by Zed, Oxford, UK.
Printed by Fine Print (Services) Ltd, Oxford, UK.

Printed with vegetable inks on fully biodegradable and
recyclable paper manufactured from sustainable forests.

Low emissions
during production

Low
chlorine

Sustainable
forests

Introduction

Psoriasis is one of the most common clinical dermatological conditions and recent evidence points to an etiology encompassing systemic, 'immunologic', autoimmune and genetic elements. It is important to recognize that psoriasis is a term that embraces a spectrum of disease, ranging from localized plaques to more severe generalized involvement, with or without psoriatic arthritis and the associated manifestations of other autoimmune diseases. However, all patients, regardless of the severity of their condition, may suffer from a reduced quality of life, particularly in relation to work and social/personal interactions.

Fast Facts – Psoriasis reviews the differential diagnoses and outlines a practical and comprehensive approach to management. This second edition has been updated throughout and also includes two important new chapters.

In Chapter 8, Dr Laura Winterfield (Department of Dermatology, University of Texas, Southwestern Medical School, Dallas) summarizes the role of the so-called biological therapies. Advances in our knowledge of the immunologic events in psoriasis, together with modern biotechnology, have led to the development of these highly selective therapies, which aim to modulate or block specific aspects of the many complex immunologic pathways involved in disease pathogenesis. Over the past 3–4 years, these agents have played an increasingly important role in the treatment of moderate-to-severe psoriasis. It is hoped that, because of their specificity, they may be associated with fewer side effects than traditional treatments.

In Chapter 9, Professor Philip Mease (Head of Seattle Rheumatology Associates, Chief of Rheumatology Clinical Research at the Swedish Hospital Medical Center, Seattle, and Clinical Professor at the University of Washington School of Medicine, Seattle) describes the clinical presentation and management of psoriatic arthritis, which results in substantial morbidity for a proportion of patients with psoriasis.

Epidemiology

Psoriasis is a common chronic inflammatory skin disease that affects approximately 2% of the population. Although all races are affected, there is considerable interracial variation. For example, psoriasis is relatively common in white people, but appears to be very uncommon in native American Indians and in Japanese people. Prevalence appears to be highest in Scandinavian countries and northern Europe. Men and women are affected equally. The usual age of onset is 20–35 years, with 75% of all cases occurring for the first time before the age of 40 years. However, psoriasis can occur at any age.

Based on age of onset, human leukocyte antigen (HLA) association and disease course, two types of chronic plaque psoriasis have been described.

- Type I, the commonest form, occurs in young adults with a high probability of a positive family history. Affected individuals tend to have more severe disease that runs a more irregular course.
- Type II psoriasis has a peak incidence between 50 and 60 years of age. In these individuals, a positive family history is very uncommon and the disease tends to be mild and localized.

Approximately 80% of patients with type I psoriasis are HLA-Cw6 positive, compared with only 20% of those with type II psoriasis.

Although psoriasis is rarely fatal, it severely affects a patient's quality of life, in terms of both psychological and physical well-being. Studies comparing psoriasis with other important chronic diseases have shown that the impact of psoriasis on the patient's quality of life is at least as great as that of ischemic heart disease, diabetes and chronic obstructive airways disease. Psoriasis is therefore a disease of major socioeconomic importance; in the USA alone, the annual cost to society has been estimated at US$3 billion.

In the UK, although the majority of psoriasis patients have relatively mild disease, current evidence suggests that 30% require second-line treatment (phototherapy or systemic medication) that involves referral to a dermatologist and perhaps 40% of all dermatology inpatients have psoriasis. In the USA, where inpatient dermatology care is rarely available, and also at many institutions in the UK, specialized psoriasis day centers have evolved for patients with moderate-to-severe disease.

Genetics. In 1963, Gunnar Lomholtz, a pioneer in the epidemiology of psoriasis, stated in his classic thesis that the disease 'is capricious and refuses to part with its innermost secret', but also wrote: 'that psoriasis is genetically conditioned is beyond doubt'. The validity of this statement has been borne out by population, family and twin studies, which all suggest an important genetic component to the disease.

The role of genetic predisposition in determining whether an individual develops psoriasis is at least as great as in many other chronic inflammatory diseases, including inflammatory bowel disease and multiple sclerosis. Many investigators are now using modern molecular genetics technology to try to unravel the genes that cause psoriasis. Such studies hold great promise for the development of highly specific treatments and new diagnostic and prognostic aids.

Numerous chromosomal loci have been discovered for psoriasis (Figure 1.1). However, only 30% of patients have a family history of the disease and it is not yet known how psoriasis is inherited. In some families, psoriasis appears to behave like a Mendelian autosomal dominant disease, whereas in other cases there is little or no family history. It has been suggested that psoriasis may represent a spectrum of diseases in which different genes, working either alone or in concert (polygenic disease), are important in different families.

Environmental factors also play a key etiologic role (Figure 1.1). For example, in 60% of patients with guttate psoriasis the disease was precipitated by systemic, usually upper respiratory tract, streptococcal infection. Other important environmental factors

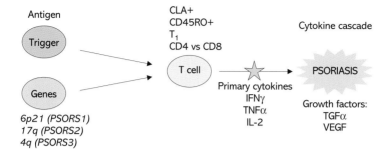

Figure 1.1 The interplay between environmental, genetic and immunologic factors that occurs in lesional skin. Antigens may be environmental antigens, superantigens or autoantigens. CLA, cutaneous lymphocyte-associated antigen; T_1, type I T-helper and T-cytotoxic cells; IFN, interferon; IL, interleukin; TGF, transforming growth factor; TNF, tumor necrosis factor; VEGF, vascular endothelial growth factor.

include drugs, particularly lithium and antimalarials, and physical or psychological stress. Excessive alcohol intake is also associated with disease deterioration and makes management more difficult.

Pathophysiology

Psoriasis is characterized by bright red, elevated, scaly plaques. These clinical features mirror the characteristic pathophysiological events that occur in lesional skin.

Epidermal hyperproliferation. There is an increase in the number of proliferating keratinocytes in the basal layer of the epidermis. This, together with loss of differentiation, is responsible for the thick, silvery scale seen clinically. The growth rate of the psoriatic epidermis is up to 10 times that of normal epidermis.

Expansion of the dermal vasculature. The blood vessels in the upper dermis become dilated and hyperpermeable, and actively increase in number. This expansion of the dermal vasculature accounts for the vivid red color of active plaques.

Accumulation of inflammatory cells. These cells – neutrophils and T lymphocytes in particular – accumulate in both the dermal and epidermal layers of the skin.

Primary pathophysiological event. Which of the factors described above represents the primary pathophysiological event has been debated for more than 100 years. In 1896, Radcliffe Crocker, a famous 19th-century English dermatologist, stated that two theories could account for the development of psoriasis: 'First, inflammation in the dermis is the primary event and hyperplasia the secondary; the second, inflammatory changes in the dermis are a secondary event.' Debate persists today. Most evidence indicates that lymphocytes play a key role in the disease process, and that the epidermal proliferation and loss of differentiation are secondary, a consequence of the release of mediators from infiltrating lymphocytes. Indeed, it has been postulated that psoriasis is an autoimmune disease. The observation of an increased prevalence of psoriasis among patients with other organ-specific inflammatory diseases, such as ulcerative colitis and Crohn's disease, is consistent with this hypothesis.

Immunologic aspects. Evidence that psoriasis is primarily an immunologic disease comes from many different sources. In evolving lesions, lymphocytes infiltrate early into the skin, prior to epidermal and other changes. Psoriasis is associated with certain HLA antigens, particularly HLA-Cw6 and HLA-B57, which are cell-surface molecules critical to the regulation of T-lymphocyte function. Experimentally, psoriasis can be induced in non-lesional skin transplanted onto mice by injection of lymphocytes from the same patient. Finally, psoriasis responds rapidly to treatments designed to inhibit T lymphocyte function, such as ciclosporin (cyclosporin).

Considerable progress has been made in identifying the precise lymphocytes that cause the disease. However, the antigens – foreign or auto – to which these lymphocytes are responding are currently unknown.

These experimental findings are key to our understanding of psoriasis. They are also of considerable clinical importance, as the majority of drugs in clinical development are targeted specifically at modulating lymphocyte activity in skin (immunotherapy).

Key points – epidemiology and pathophysiology

- Psoriasis affects approximately 2% of the population; however, there is considerable interracial variation in prevalence.
- The usual age of onset is 20–35 years.
- There is a family history of psoriasis in 30% of patients.
- There is growing evidence that psoriasis is primarily an immunologic T-cell-driven disease.
- Important environmental triggers include infection, drugs, and physical and psychological stress.
- Three key events characterize the pathophysiology of psoriasis: epidermal hyperproliferation, angiogenesis and accumulation of inflammatory cells.
- The impact of psoriasis on the patient's quality of life is similar – physically and emotionally – to that of ischemic heart disease, diabetes or chronic obstructive airways disease.

Key references

Barker JNWN. The pathophysiology of psoriasis. *Lancet* 1991;338:227–30.

Bowcock AM, Barker JN. Genetics of psoriasis: the potential impact on new therapies. *J Am Acad Dermatol* 2003;49(2 suppl):S51–6.

Christophers E. Psoriasis – epidemiology and clinical spectrum. *Clin Exp Dermatol* 2001;26:314–20.

Chronic plaque psoriasis (psoriasis vulgaris) accounts for approximately 85% of all cases of psoriasis. The majority of patients develop clinical signs of psoriasis before the age of 35 years, with about 10% of patients developing the condition during childhood. A history of long-standing 'dandruff', scaling in the ears, pruritus ani or vulvae, arthralgias or the presence of other autoimmune diseases, such as inflammatory bowel disease, diabetes or thyroid disease, may be clues to a diagnosis of psoriasis (Table 2.1). There is no blood test specific to psoriasis.

TABLE 2.1

Important factors in the patient's history

Medical history
- Persistent scaling in the ears
- Concomitant or previously diagnosed autoimmune disease
- Joint problems
- Long-standing 'dandruff'
- Pruritus ani or vulvae

Family history
- Psoriasis
- Rheumatoid disease

Precipitating factors
- Antecedent infections (particularly streptococcal)
- Physical trauma
- Emotional or metabolic stress

Drugs likely to exacerbate psoriasis
- Antimalarials (e.g. chloroquine)
- Interferons
- Lithium
- Systemic glucocorticoids

Clinical manifestations

Psoriasis exhibits a range of histological features (Figure 2.1 and Table 2.2). All lesions show varying degrees of three cardinal characteristics:

- scaling
- thickening (induration)
- inflammation (redness).

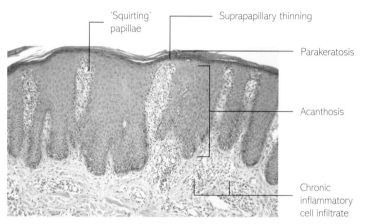

Figure 2.1 A photomicrograph showing the typical histological features of psoriasis (magnification: x 40).

TABLE 2.2

Histological features of psoriasis

- Acanthosis: thickening of the epidermis
- Parakeratosis: retention of nuclei in the stratum corneum
- Suprapapillary thinning: only a few layers of epidermal cells are observed above the dermal papillae
- Papillary elongation: increased lengthening of the papillary folds
- Increased prominence of the papillary vasculature
- 'Squirting' papillae: neutrophils noted in the dermal papillae and frequently in the adjacent epidermis. This may even produce microabscesses in the more inflammatory or pustular variants
- Chronic perivascular inflammatory response noted in the dermis

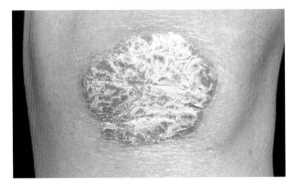

Figure 2.2 Typical plaque of chronic psoriasis showing discoid configuration, thick adherent scale, induration and redness.

The classic symmetry, silvery scale and vivid reddish-purple color (Figure 2.2) allow psoriasis to be easily differentiated from other skin disorders in the majority of cases.

Shape of lesions. Classically, a psoriatic lesion is oval-shaped (discoid) (Figures 2.2 and 2.3), although atypical lesions featuring

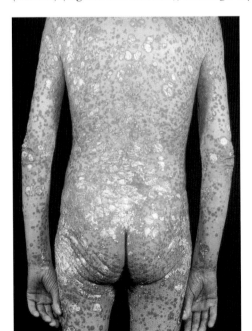

Figure 2.3 Extensive chronic plaque psoriasis.

linear, annular or geographic 'map-like' configurations may be present. Other morphological variants, which can coexist in one patient, include:

- guttate lesions (predominantly on the trunk)
- flexural forms (body folds)
- erythrodermic psoriasis (total body erythema and scaling)
- pustular psoriasis (localized or generalized)
- localized variants, such as palmar–plantar forms.

Guttate lesions, approximately 1 cm in diameter, often follow a streptococcal infection in younger patients. Multiple 'drop-like' lesions occur (Figure 2.4) and are typically distributed on the trunk; they may develop rapidly over a period of a week. Larger plaques may be seen in areas such as the lumbar–sacral region, and frequently involve the natal cleft with extension to perianal areas.

Flexural forms (inverse psoriasis), commonly seen in obese patients, occur in normal body folds, such as under the breasts, and in the inguinal and axillary regions (Figure 2.5).

Erythrodermic psoriasis is relatively uncommon. It involves the entire body surface and may be precipitated by inappropriate use of systemic glucocorticoids, infections or even phototherapy or sunburn. Patients are febrile, and often have high white-cell counts and problems with temperature control. Associated ankle edema is common. Frequently, cardiac and renal decompensation is seen, particularly in the elderly.

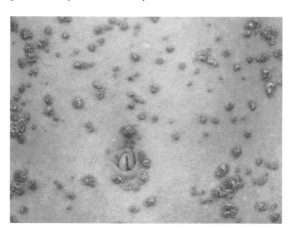

Figure 2.4 Typical guttate psoriasis, with multiple 'drop-like' lesions on the trunk.

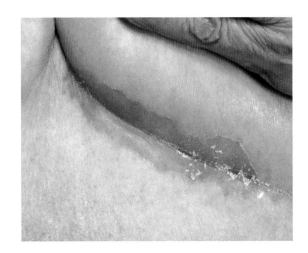

Figure 2.5
Flexural psoriasis beneath the breast. Note the absence of scale and the livid red color.

Pustular psoriasis can appear as two forms. The first form occurs in association with erythrodermic psoriasis, in which multiple tiny pustules, with or without coalescence, are scattered throughout the inflamed body surface. The second is a more localized form in which multiple small pustules, often on an erythematous and hyperkeratotic base, are present on the palms and soles (Figure 2.6); this is sometimes referred to as palmar–plantar pustulosis.

Distribution of psoriatic lesions is highly symmetrical in most cases, except when modified, for example, by chronic scratching on the back or sides of the scalp. Regions commonly involved include the thicker areas of the skin, such as the scalp, elbows, knees, sacral area and knuckles on the hand dorsa. Although psoriasis is normally considered to be a non-itchy condition, the majority of patients quickly develop the habit of scratching, leading to a marked increase in thickening (lichenification) of individual plaques. Similarly, day-to-day trauma may modify lesions in areas such as the hands and feet.

Secondary candidiasis in body folds can also modify psoriasis, as can concurrent disease such as human immunodeficiency virus (HIV) infection, which frequently results in a more inflammatory form of psoriasis, often with severe facial involvement.

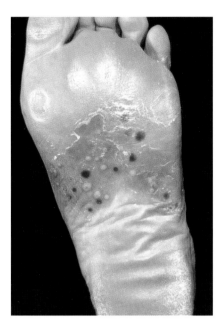

Figure 2.6 Localized, chronic pustular psoriasis involving the sole of the foot. Multiple sterile, yellow pustules occur, which evolve into brown macules and subsequently desquamate.

Color of lesions. Psoriasis lesions are usually a more vivid purplish-red color than most other dermatoses, such as eczema. Even in early lesions, gentle scratching of the affected skin will elicit the classic silvery scale. Gentle detachment of the overlying silvery scale will produce fine, pinpoint bleeding on the surface of the skin; this is known as the Auspitz sign and is highly diagnostic.

Sites of disease involvement
For diagnosis, the whole body surface should be evaluated. Similarly, the total skin area should be assessed when deciding on appropriate treatment.

Scalp involvement may range from a moderate degree of silvery scale, resembling seborrheic dermatitis, to thick well-circumscribed plaques covering major portions of the scalp surface (Figure 2.7). The patient's habitual scratching will often modify the psoriasis to produce asymmetric plaques, particularly on the sides and the posterior scalp. Extension beyond the scalp fringes onto the forehead, temples, sideburns and nape of the neck is common.

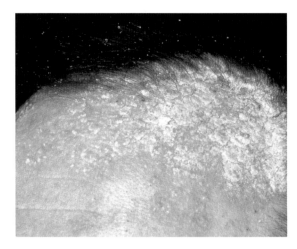

Figure 2.7 Plaque psoriasis involving the scalp margin. Chronic scalp scaling may cause significant embarrassment to the patient.

Ears. The retroauricular folds, which extend into the scalp margin, are a common site of involvement, often producing secondary fissuring. Psoriasis is also one of the most common causes of otitis externa, with a classic silvery scale on an erythematous base extending into the ear canal (Figure 2.8). Wafting of the scale down the ear canal may produce a pseudo-membrane, which may impair hearing with time.

Face. Involvement of the face is not uncommon. Scaling, erythema and even plaque formation may be noted in the eyebrows, together with scaly erythema around the sides of the nose, scalp and sideburn fringes, which extends onto the forehead and temple regions (Figure 2.9). In addition, men frequently develop psoriasis within the beard region, particularly the sides of the neck, because of shaving trauma.

Trunk. Individual discoid plaques are usually seen in this region (see Figure 2.3). There is great variation in size and shape, but larger plaques are often noted in the lumbar–sacral area. Involvement of the umbilicus and gluteal cleft is common. Lesions in the folds of the breasts are also common – usually the classic silvery scale is not seen, but a distinct erythema is present (see Figure 2.5). In the flexures, secondary candidiasis, with development of pustules peripheral to the well-demarcated erythematous areas, is a common sequela.

Extremities. Localized discoid plaques are common on the elbows and knees. Symmetrical discoid plaques, ranging in size and number, are particularly prominent on the distal portions of the extremities, particularly the shins and ulnar surface of the arms.

Hands and feet. Two main forms of psoriasis occur at these sites.

- The hyperkeratotic variant has localized well-circumscribed or more diffuse erythematous silvery plaques, with or without fissures. There is frequent involvement of the palmar surface (Figure 2.10) and sides of the fingers.
- The pustular variant (see Figure 2.6) has multiple tiny pustules (0.1–0.3 cm in diameter), with or without associated erythema,

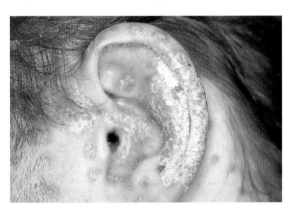

Figure 2.8 Plaque psoriasis affecting the ear and encroaching onto the external auditory meatus. Note the sideburn involvement.

Figure 2.9 Extension of scalp involvement onto the forehead (as here) and temples is common.

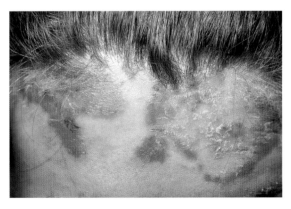

scaling or crusting of the intervening skin. These pustules are sterile and are caused by accumulation of polymorphonuclear leukocytes within the epidermis.

Genitalia are frequently involved. In men, a well-circumscribed, thin, erythematous lesion is seen on the glans penis, usually with minimal associated silvery scale because of the thinness of the skin in this region. In women, a similar, well-circumscribed, purplish-red erythema is noted enveloping the vaginal opening. The pubic region is often involved in both sexes. Direct extension of disease from the natal cleft may involve perianal skin and cause pruritus ani.

Nails. Involvement of the nails can take several forms.

Pitting describes discrete, well-circumscribed depressions of about 1 mm in diameter on the nail surface. This may involve only a few nails or the majority of the fingernails and, to a lesser degree, the toenails.

Onycholysis is a separation of the nail from the nail bed at its free edge. It produces a white to yellowish discoloration of the distal nail plate, ranging from 1–2 mm at the distal free edge to involvement of the entire nail (Figure 2.11).

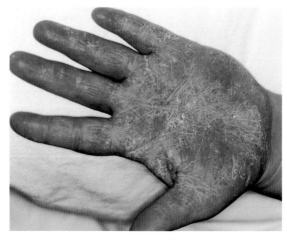

Figure 2.10 Hyperkeratotic plaque psoriasis affecting the palm. Distinction from tinea manum and chronic hand eczema may be extremely difficult.

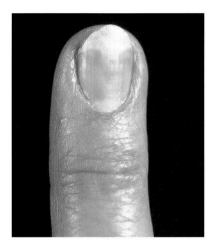

Figure 2.11 Onycholysis (loosening of the nail from the underlying nail bed) with adjacent pink–red color change known as the 'oil-drop sign'.

Subungual hyperkeratosis. Silvery white crusting and debris are seen underneath the free edge of the nail in association with some degree of thickening of the nail plate (Figure 2.12).

'Oil-drop sign' refers to the well-circumscribed, usually circular, light pink-to-red color change seen on the surface of the nail, separate and distinct from onycholysis (see Figure 2.11).

Koebner phenomenon, also known as isomorphic response, describes induction of psoriasis as a result of trauma at sites of previous non-involvement. It occurs at scratches, surgical incisions

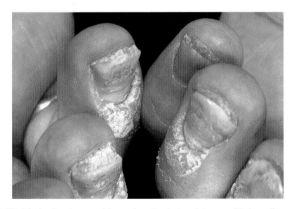

Figure 2.12 Marked subungual hyperkeratosis involving multiple nails; note also periungual psoriasis.

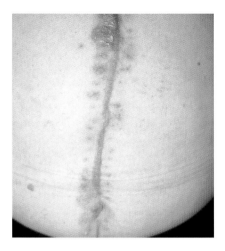

Figure 2.13 Multiple patches of psoriasis occurring in a surgical scar (Koebner phenomenon).

(Figure 2.13), body-piercing sites and scars, and with friction from clothing or jewellery, such as rings, watches and earrings.

Psoriatic joint disease

On clinical and radiological evaluation, approximately 25% of patients have confirmed psoriatic arthritis. Many more complain of mild arthralgias.

Five major patterns of psoriatic arthritis are recognized, with overlapping clinical expressions frequently seen:

• distal interphalangeal involvement (Figure 2.14)

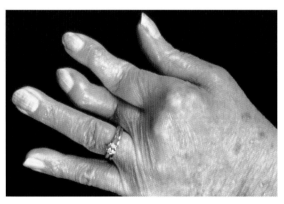

Figure 2.14 Small joint psoriatic arthropathy involving proximal and distal interphalangeal joints, some with marked joint destruction (arthritis mutilans).

- symmetrical polyarthritis, indistinguishable from rheumatoid arthritis
- asymmetrical oligoarthritis
- psoriatic spondylarthropathy
- arthritis mutilans, a rare variant that is most likely to affect the hands and feet (see Figure 2.14).

Patients with the most common form – distal interphalangeal disease – frequently have concomitant nail disease, often localized to the same digits as the joint disease.

Key points – clinical presentation

- Medical history, family history and physical examination are all important in establishing the diagnosis of psoriasis.
- Psoriasis is a clinical diagnosis; there is no blood test specific for this disease.
- Chronic discoid plaque psoriasis is the most common subtype of psoriasis.
- The scalp, elbows, knees and sacrum are the areas most commonly affected by psoriasis.
- Psoriasis can sometimes be triggered by infection, trauma, stress or medications.

Key references

Abel EA, DiCicco LM, Orenberg EK et al. Drugs in exacerbation of psoriasis. *J Am Acad Dermatol* 1986;15:1007–22.

Boyd AS, Menter A. Erythrodermic psoriasis. Precipitating factors, course, and prognosis in 50 patients. *J Am Acad Dermatol* 1989;21:985–91.

Chalmers RR, O'Sullivan T, Owen CC, Griffiths CC. A systematic review of treatments for guttate psoriasis. *Br J Dermatol* 2001;145:891–4.

Champion RH, Burton JL, Burns DA, Breathnach SM. *Textbook of Dermatology.* London: Blackwell Science, 1998:1597–1607.

Farber EM, Nall L. Nail psoriasis. *Cutis* 1992;50:174–8.

Gladman DD. Current concepts in psoriatic arthritis. *Curr Opin Rheumatol* 2002;14:361–6.

Naldi L, Peli L, Parazzini F, Carrel CF. Family history of psoriasis, stressful life events, and recent infectious disease are risk factors for a first episode of acute guttate psoriasis: results of a case-control study. *J Am Acad Dermatol* 2001;44:433–8.

Schubert C. [Inflammatory skin diseases. An assortment of clinically relevant disease conditions.] *Pathologe* 2002;23:9–19. German.

van de Kerkhof PCM. *Textbook of Psoriasis*. Oxford: Blackwell Science, 1999:3–29.

Weiss G, Shemer A, Trau H. The Koebner phenomenon: review of the literature. *J Eur Acad Dermatol Venereol* 2002;16:241–8.

Although diagnosis is relatively straightforward, a number of other dermatological entities may be confused with psoriasis (Table 3.1). A careful history and physical examination, together with laboratory findings, will usually reveal the correct diagnosis.

Infection

Candidiasis. In flexural areas, peripheral pustules are characteristic of *Candida* infection. The presence of yeast and pseudo-hyphae in Gram-stained microscopy specimens will confirm infection.

Tinea, or ringworm, is an infection caused by a dermatophyte fungus and may sometimes be mistaken for psoriasis. Where diagnostic doubt exists, appropriate mycological specimens (skin, hair and/or nail) should be taken.

Tinea capitis is ringworm of the head. Although a minor degree of hair thinning is not uncommon in established cases of psoriasis,

TABLE 3.1

Differential diagnosis of psoriasis

- Candidiasis
- Tinea infection
- Syphilis (secondary)
- Eczema (atopic or nummular)
- Contact dermatitis
- Superficial basal cell carcinoma and Bowen's disease
- Cutaneous T-cell lymphoma (mycosis fungoides)
- Pityriasis rosea

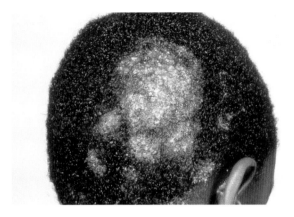

Figure 3.1 A scalp infected with *Trichophyton tonsurans* – a common cause of tinea capitis. Clinical signs vary from mild scaling to, as here, marked alopecia and suppurative inflammation (kerion formation).

well demarcated areas of hair loss and signs such as the 'black dots' or fractured hair shafts characteristic of tinea infection (Figure 3.1) are highly unusual in psoriasis. In addition, tinea capitis seldom shows the classic silvery scale of psoriasis.

Tinea corporis affects the body (Figure 3.2). Lack of symmetrical lesions, presence of peripheral scale and central clearing are all more characteristic of tinea than of psoriasis.

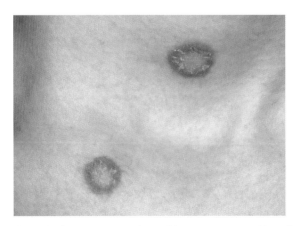

Figure 3.2 A patch of tinea corporis due to *Microsporum canis*. Note the typical peripheral scale and relative central clearing.

Tinea cruris affects the groin area, and is characterized by central clearing with an advancing edge. The lesion has a non-silvery, fine scale, particularly at the periphery, and frequently extends more on the left than the right side.

Tinea pedis is ringworm of the feet. In the vesicular form, clear vesicles are noted (in contrast to the whitish-yellow pustule of psoriasis). In the 'dry moccasin' variety of tinea pedis, a relative lack of symmetry is seen.

Tinea manum is ringworm of the hands. It presents as fine powdery scale, particularly involving the palms and palmar creases. Again, it is usually asymmetrical.

Tinea unguium infection of the nails may be extremely difficult to distinguish from psoriatic nail involvement, particularly in toenails. Furthermore, patients with psoriatic nail disease are more likely than individuals without pre-existing nail disease to have an associated fungal infection. A search for nail pits and clinical evidence of cutaneous psoriasis or tinea of the feet is important. Appropriate cultures taken from the nails are often required to make this diagnosis.

Secondary syphilis. The guttate (drop-like) forms of psoriasis may mimic secondary syphilis. Therefore, it is important to conduct a careful search for a primary syphilitic lesion, together with associated lymphadenopathy, mucosal lesions and palmar–plantar lesions with a peripheral collarette of scale, which are characteristic of secondary syphilis. If in doubt, serological testing for syphilis should be considered.

Eczema/dermatitis

Discoid eczema. Individual patches are usually more pruritic, lack a silvery scale and are less likely to show the more vivid, characteristic purplish-red color of psoriasis (Figure 3.3).

Hand and foot eczema. Hyperkeratotic forms of eczema, particularly in atopic patients, may be identical in appearance to psoriasis. Taking a skin biopsy to differentiate it from psoriasis is

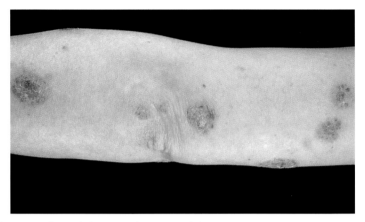

Figure 3.3 Discoid (nummular) eczema of the arm.

rarely helpful. Clues to the diagnosis include a history of atopy (hay fever and/or asthma), a lack of psoriasis elsewhere on the body, and evidence of eczema elsewhere on the skin. Clinically, psoriasis is usually more clearly demarcated than eczema, even on the palms and soles.

Flexural (atopic) eczema. A history of atopy, including asthma, allergies or rhinitis, will frequently exclude psoriasis. In addition, the lack of classic psoriatic nail involvement is important.

Contact dermatitis is seldom symmetrical and is more pruritic than psoriasis, particularly in the early stages.

Pompholyx of the palms and soles (dishydrotic eczema) may frequently mimic pustular psoriasis of the palms and soles. However, in the initial stage, pompholyx vesicles are clear (in contrast to the yellowish color of pustular psoriasis) and are intensely pruritic.

Neoplasms
Skin cancers. Individual lesions of multicentric, superficial basal cell carcinoma and Bowen's disease (squamous cell carcinoma in situ) may appear highly suggestive of psoriasis (Figure 3.4). However, these neoplasms usually occur singly or are fewer in number, are

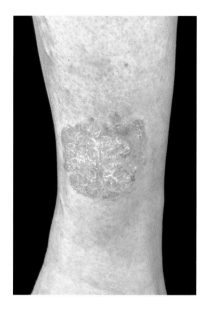

Figure 3.4 A patch of Bowen's disease on the lower leg of an elderly patient. In contrast to psoriasis, lesions are either single or few in number and are not symmetrical.

never symmetrical and do not show the classic silvery scale of psoriasis. If localized 'psoriasiform' lesions fail to respond to traditional topical therapy, this diagnosis should be considered and a skin biopsy performed.

Cutaneous T-cell lymphoma (mycosis fungoides). In its early stages, when patches or plaques are apparent, this condition may closely resemble psoriasis. Fine atrophy ('cigarette-paper wrinkling') within the lesions, plus a lack of response to traditional antipsoriatic therapy, may be useful in differentiating cutaneous T-cell lymphoma from psoriasis. However, biopsy is usually required; this may need to be repeated at intervals for confirmation.

Pityriasis rosea

Onset of pityriasis rosea is typically acute, and the first sign is usually a single large 'herald patch' presenting a few days before the characteristic truncal rash. This is normally self-limiting over a period 8–12 weeks, producing multiple oval scaly lesions in a 'Christmas tree' distribution (Figure 3.5). Distinction from acute guttate psoriasis may be difficult.

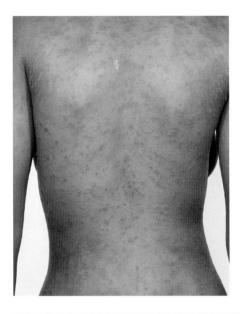

Figure 3.5 Pityriasis rosea, showing the multiple red scaly plaques that typically occur in a 'Christmas tree' distribution on the trunk, following the rib lines.

Key points – differential diagnosis

- Various dermatological disorders can resemble psoriasis, including other inflammatory dermatoses, infections and neoplasms.
- Usually, routine history together with physical examination and laboratory findings will reveal the correct diagnosis.

Key references

Champion RH, Burton JL, Burns DA, Breathnach SM. *Textbook of Dermatology.* London: Blackwell Science, 1998:1597–1608.

Elmer KB, George RM. Cutaneous T-cell lymphoma presenting as benign dermatoses. *Am Fam Physician* 1999;59:2809–13.

Eslick GD. Atypical pityriasis rosea or psoriasis guttata? Early examination is the key to a correct diagnosis. *Int J Dermatol* 2002;41:788–91.

Successful management of psoriasis in the primary care setting requires clinical experience and ready access to specialist dermatological advice, nursing expertise and, when necessary, hospital-based dermatology treatment centers.

The overall goals of any treatment program for psoriasis must be to:
- improve the patient's quality of life
- achieve long-term remission and disease control
- reduce individual drug toxicity
- carefully evaluate individual treatments and monitor their cost-effectiveness.

Initial consultation

In the USA, approximately 50% of patients with psoriasis are not under the care of a physician, probably because of:
- frustration at a lack of understanding and insight into this highly visible, chronic disease
- failure of available therapies to maintain adequate remission
- physicians' lack of planning/time spent with patients in consultation and discussion.

Precise data are not available for the UK, but similar sentiments have been documented. Most patients with psoriasis will present to their primary care physician, but only 20–30% of psoriasis patients in the UK will be referred to a dermatologist.

It is important that physicians discuss the chronic, relapsing, non-contagious, benign nature of psoriasis with patients to reassure them and improve their understanding of the condition. Many patients who present with mild psoriasis do not necessarily want active therapy – a diagnosis and reassurance may be sufficient, particularly given that available treatments do not alter the natural history or activity of the disease. Excellent educational support material and resources are available for both patients and physicians from the Psoriasis Association in the UK and the National Psoriasis Foundation in the USA (see Useful addresses, page 99).

The aspects of psoriasis that trouble the patient most should be determined. Notably, the degree to which psoriasis affects a person's daily life does not necessarily correlate with objective scores of disease severity. Questionnaires designed to quantify these issues, such as Finlay's quality of life index, can provide a useful insight into a patient's perception of his or her disease and help to tailor individual therapy.

Factors in the patient's social history can contribute to disease severity or affect treatment outcome and, although sometimes difficult to change, it is important to recognize such factors in the overall disease management. Lifestyle advice regarding the benefits of exercise, avoiding excess alcohol intake and following a healthy diet may be useful. However, despite multiple claims, no one specific diet has been shown to be more beneficial than another. Patients should be advised to avoid trauma, friction and scratching (including shaving trauma in men and women, scratching of ear canals, harsh shampooing and picking of crusts on the scalp). In addition, providing information about stress reduction and management is often of value.

Psoriasis may be exacerbated by systemic drugs, such as antimalarials, taken for other problems (see Table 2.1, page 12); if feasible, medication should be altered. Finally, treatment of coexisting illnesses, particularly acute respiratory infections in younger patients, is important to reduce the risk of an acute flare-up of pre-existing psoriasis.

Available treatments
Treatments available for psoriasis include a wide range of topical therapies, phototherapy (including photochemotherapy, see Chapter 5) and a variety of systemic agents, some with potentially significant side effects (see Chapter 6). Many factors influence the choice of therapy for an individual (Table 4.1). Approximately 70% of patients with psoriasis can be managed using topical therapy alone.

TABLE 4.1

Factors to consider when treating psoriasis patients

- Patient's perception of disease severity
- Objective measures of the pattern, extent and severity of disease
- Amount of time the patient is able to devote to therapy
- Previous treatments for psoriasis
- Coexistent medical problems
- Other drug therapy

Before beginning therapy, the patient should have a realistic expectation of the outcome. In practice, this means explaining that treatment will be lengthy and is not curative, and that the psoriasis is likely to relapse if therapy is discontinued. In addition, it is crucial to spend sufficient time explaining practical aspects, such as:

- precisely what a treatment is designed to achieve and how
- where and for how long therapy should be applied
- any local side effects, such as irritation, staining or smell.

Detailed information about the practicalities of using the various topical agents is probably best provided by a nurse with dermatology training, though this resource is not universally available.

Chronic plaque psoriasis

In general, patients with mild-to-moderate chronic plaque psoriasis, who comprise the majority of those seeking treatment, can be managed successfully with topical agents alone. Those with more extensive chronic plaque disease may also benefit from topical therapy, though the logistics of application become difficult and more time-consuming.

A large number of different topical preparations are available (Table 4.2); topical corticosteroids and vitamin D_3 analogs are considered first-line therapy for most patients. When deciding which product to prescribe, therapeutic efficacy must be balanced against the cosmetic acceptability and the local side-effect profile, particularly as most treatments take several weeks to work.

TABLE 4.2

Topical therapies for chronic plaque psoriasis

Agent	Efficacy	Relapse rate	Side effects	Cosmetic problems
Emollients	+	+	–	+
Keratolytics	+	+	+	+
Coal-tar	++	+	+	++
Dithranol	+++	+	+	++
Corticosteroids (potent/very potent)	+++	++	++	–
Vitamin D$_3$ analogs	+++	+	+	–
Tazarotene	++	+	++	+

–, little or none; +++, very great or frequent (or in the case of side effects and cosmetic problems, severe).
Adapted with permission from Greaves M, Weinstein G. Treatment of psoriasis. *N Engl J Med* 1995;332:581–8. Copyright © 1995 Massachusetts Medical Society. All rights reserved.

Previous therapy. Tried and tested treatments that the patient has previously found helpful are likely to be the best choice again. However, patients commonly cite previous therapy as unhelpful, so it is important to establish the reasons for this and the way in which the treatment failed. Sometimes expectations are unrealistic; if the patient was hoping for a cure, he will be disappointed if his psoriasis relapses off therapy. Always ensure that the treatment duration has been adequate. For example, calcipotriol and tazarotene therapy needs to be continued for 8–12 weeks to achieve maximum benefit. Frequently, local side effects and poor cosmetic acceptability are the reasons for patient dissatisfaction with previous therapy. These may be overcome by using a different formulation of the active ingredient or changing the frequency or time of application.

Choice of formulation. Active agents may be available as a lotion, water-miscible cream and/or ointment. Choice of formulation and type of therapy will depend on both patient preference and the site/pattern of psoriasis. For plaque psoriasis on the body, ointments are preferable owing to their emollient properties and lack of sensitizers. Creams are suitable for use at flexural sites and, because they are less greasy than ointments, are often prescribed for the face. Lotions are appropriate for hairy areas. Irritant preparations, such as dithranol, are unsuitable for very inflammatory, weeping or eroded areas of psoriasis, but are entirely appropriate for thick, hyperkeratotic disease.

Patient motivation. Some patients are unlikely to apply therapy more than once a day on a regular basis; others may be willing and able to spend a significant amount of time applying treatments. A well motivated patient, with adequate bathing facilities, time and perhaps someone to help with topical applications, will cope with a home-use, short-contact dithranol regimen together with emollients and topical corticosteroids or a vitamin D or A analog. However, other patients would find this unacceptable. Such variations in patient acceptability should be taken into account when prescribing.

Emollients. According to the classic textbook description, psoriasis does not itch. However, a recent survey suggests that itching is a prominent and troublesome symptom in more than 60% of patients with psoriasis. Regular use of an emollient, particularly in colder months, can alleviate pruritus, reduce scale and enhance penetration of concomitant topical therapy.

Keratolytic agents. Agents such as salicylic acid and urea are often included in topical psoriasis preparations; they reduce scale and enhance penetration of other active agents.

Topical corticosteroids
Mode of action. Corticosteroids possess marked anti-inflammatory, antiproliferative and immunomodulatory properties that may be relevant to their efficacy in psoriasis. However, their precise mode of action is unknown.

Efficacy. Topical corticosteroids vary in anti-inflammatory activity. The *British National Formulary* cites four groups (mild, moderate, potent and very potent) based on the ability of the steroid molecule to blanch human skin in the vasoconstrictor assay. In the USA, seven groups of corticosteroid potency are recognized (group I being the most potent), based on the vasoconstrictor assay and/or clinical effectiveness in psoriasis.

Potent and very potent topical corticosteroids (groups I–V in the US system) are extremely effective for chronic plaque psoriasis on the trunk, limbs and scalp, with clearance of plaques after 1–2 weeks of therapy. For the face and flexural sites, mild (group VII) corticosteroids are effective; corticosteroids of moderate potency (group VI) should be used at these sites rarely and only for short periods.

Continuous use of corticosteroids, particularly potent and very potent agents, may lead to loss of efficacy (known as tachyphylaxis) and an increased risk of significant local side effects, such as cutaneous atrophy. On stopping therapy, severe rebound or even pustular psoriasis may develop. Despite these hazards, corticosteroids form an important component of topical therapy for chronic plaque psoriasis.

Various measures have been adopted to reduce the incidence of side effects while retaining therapeutic efficacy. These include:

- using the least potent corticosteroid required to control disease
- applying the agent once daily
- giving intermittent pulses of therapy (e.g. at weekends) once remission has been induced
- diluting the corticosteroid and/or combining it with other active agents, such as coal-tar, dithranol or salicylic acid, in a single preparation (however, the potency, and thus efficacy, of the corticosteroid in these preparations may be unpredictable, particularly in non-proprietary products)
- combining the corticosteroid with other non-steroidal topical therapies, such as calcipotriol or tazarotene (see pages 38–42 and 45–46, respectively).

Side effects, safety and cosmetic acceptability. Topical corticosteroids are popular with patients, and remain first-line therapy in the USA, because of their immediate efficacy and excellent cosmetic acceptability. Therefore, it is important for physicians to outline the problems associated with continuous, long-term therapy and to monitor prescriptions carefully to avoid excessive use.

Local side effects include:
- skin atrophy and telangiectasia (usually reversible)
- skin bleaching, particularly in those with darker skin tones (reversible)
- striae (irreversible) (Figure 4.1)
- masking of local infection (rarely a problem in psoriasis)
- rapid relapse or rebound of psoriasis on stopping therapy
- transformation of stable plaque psoriasis to pustular psoriasis
- tachyphylaxis (mechanism unknown).

Rarely, significant percutaneous absorption of corticosteroid may occur, leading to pituitary–adrenal axis suppression and Cushing's syndrome. Infants and children are at particular risk because of their large surface-area-to-volume ratio. Newer corticosteroids, such as mometasone and fluticasone, are rapidly inactivated or metabolized following percutaneous absorption, and may be less likely to lead to significant systemic absorption.

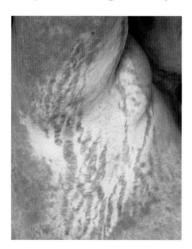

Figure 4.1 Multiple striae in a patient after inappropriate use of potent corticosteroids for flexural psoriasis.

The likelihood of corticosteroid side effects increases with potency, the total amount applied per day and the duration of treatment. The face and flexures are particularly vulnerable to local problems. Use of occlusion or addition of certain excipients, such as propylene glycol, that are designed to improve penetration and efficacy may also increase the risk of local side effects. Allergic contact dermatitis may complicate the use of topical corticosteroids and is most frequently caused by one of the excipients present in the formulation. Rarely, patients may exhibit sensitivity to the corticosteroid molecule itself.

Adherence to treatment guidelines may help to minimize the risk of local and systemic side effects (Table 4.3 and Figure 4.2).

Vitamin D$_3$ analogs

Vitamin D analogs are used widely, particularly in the UK and Europe, where they are considered first-line treatment for stable chronic plaque psoriasis.

Mode of action. Some of the effects of these agents are mediated via specific binding to the vitamin D$_3$ receptor, while others are

TABLE 4.3

Treatment guidelines to minimize side effects of corticosteroids

- No topical corticosteroid should be used regularly for more than 4 weeks without critical review

- Potent or very potent steroids (groups I–V) should not be used daily for more than 10 days; patients should be under the supervision of a dermatologist

- Patients using topical corticosteroids should have their treatment reviewed regularly, at least every 3 months

- Less than 100 g moderate potency or higher potency preparation should be used per month

- The 'finger-tip measure' may help patients to apply corticosteroids in appropriate amounts (Figure 4.2), although some argue that this may in fact lead to underuse of corticosteroids

- Corticosteroids should be used alternately with non-steroidal therapies

Use the adult finger-tip unit as your guide

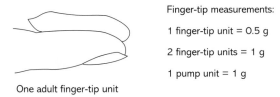

Finger-tip measurements:

1 finger-tip unit = 0.5 g

2 finger-tip units = 1 g

1 pump unit = 1 g

One adult finger-tip unit

Topical corticosteroids: single application requirements

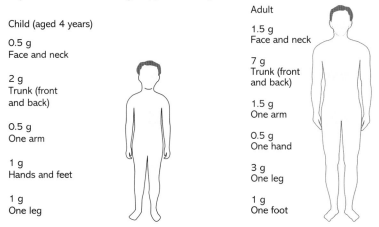

Child (aged 4 years)

0.5 g
Face and neck

2 g
Trunk (front and back)

0.5 g
One arm

1 g
Hands and feet

1 g
One leg

Adult

1.5 g
Face and neck

7 g
Trunk (front and back)

1.5 g
One arm

0.5 g
One hand

3 g
One leg

1 g
One foot

Figure 4.2 Finger-tip guidance for application of corticosteroids. Adapted with permission from Long CC, Finlay A. *Clin Exp Dermatol* 1991;16:444–8.

non-receptor-mediated. The events that contribute to the therapeutic efficacy of vitamin D$_3$ analogs in psoriasis include:

- inhibition of keratinocyte proliferation
- enhancement of normal keratinization
- inhibition of accumulation of inflammatory cells, particularly neutrophils and T lymphocytes.

Efficacy. Calcipotriol and the more recently introduced tacalcitol and calcitriol (neither licensed in the USA) are all effective in chronic plaque psoriasis and can induce significant clearing of disease after 4–6 weeks (Table 4.4). Placebo-controlled studies of these agents suggest there is little to choose between them in terms of overall efficacy. However, data from the few trials that directly

TABLE 4.4

Vitamin D_3 analogs

Formulations	Frequency of application	Maximum dose	Site of application (licensed)
Calcipotriol			
Ointment, cream, scalp application	Once or twice daily	100 g/week	Avoid face and flexures
Tacalcitol			
Ointment	Once daily	10 g/day	All sites
Calcitriol			
Ointment	Twice daily	30 g/day (applied to maximum of 35% body surface area)	All sites

compare the efficacy of these agents suggest a marginal advantage for calcipotriol (applied twice daily) over tacalcitol (once daily) and calcitriol (twice daily). All have efficacy comparable to mid-to-high-potency topical corticosteroids. Calcipotriol has also been found to be more effective and better tolerated than short-contact, home-use dithranol and tar (up to 15%). Long-term studies of calcipotriol and tacalcitol conducted for almost a year show no evidence of tachyphylaxis or significant local side effects.

The potency of calcipotriol can be increased if it is applied under occlusion or more frequently. This approach may be useful, particularly if large areas of psoriasis require treatment, although there will be an associated increase in the risk of hypercalcemia.

Although vitamin D_3 analogs are cosmetically acceptable and relatively free of side effects, their onset of action is slow compared with topical corticosteroids. However, treatment with topical corticosteroids alone carries a significant risk of skin atrophy, tachyphylaxis and severe rebound psoriasis on stopping therapy. Recent studies have shown that combination therapy with corticosteroid and calcipotriol can be used to circumvent these problems. Response rates may be increased if calcipotriol is used in the morning and a potent corticosteroid in the evening. Dovobet®, a combination preparation containing calcipotriol and betamethasone dipropionate (0.5 mg/g), recently licensed in Europe, may be useful in this regard. Alternatively, a short course (2 weeks) of a potent or very potent corticosteroid (groups I–V) can be used to induce a rapid remission, which may be maintained using calcipotriol either alone or in combination with a more moderate corticosteroid.

Calcipotriol, calcitriol and tacalcitol have also been used in combination with phototherapy (see Chapter 5) and other systemic agents. The main benefit of such combinations is a reduction in total cumulative exposure to the systemic agent or phototherapy used.

Side effects, safety and cosmetic acceptability. Calcipotriol is licensed in the UK, USA and other countries for use in children over the age of 6 years, and is effective and well tolerated in this group. Calcipotriol, tacalcitol and calcitriol are odorless and colorless, and do not stain the skin.

Local skin irritation occurs in up to 20% of patients using calcipotriol, but only rarely requires withdrawal of therapy. The more recently developed agents, tacalcitol and calcitriol, may be slightly less irritant. For example, long-term safety studies of tacalcitol report skin irritation in about 15% of patients, even though all sites were treated, compared with rates of 20% for calcipotriol where face and flexural sites were excluded. A direct comparison between calcipotriol and calcitriol used on sensitive sites (face, flexural areas and genitalia) also revealed greater tolerability with calcitriol.

Combination with a topical corticosteroid may help if local irritation is a prominent symptom. Allergic contact dermatitis occasionally complicates use of these compounds. However, sensitivity to calcipotriol, for example, does not necessarily predict sensitivity to tacalcitol.

The maximum weekly dose of calcipotriol for children aged 6–12 years is 50 g, and 75 g for those aged 12 years or more. Adults exceeding the manufacturer's recommended doses of these agents (see Table 4.4), particularly those with erythrodermic psoriasis, run the risk of hypercalcemia; 200–300 g/week predictably will increase urinary and serum calcium and depress parathyroid hormone levels.

Coal-tar is produced by destructive distillation of coal. The exact composition of coal-tar depends on the temperature during the distillation process and the type of coal used.

A variety of products is available, though reliable supplies have become difficult to obtain in some areas because of declining use and renewed concern about the oncogenic potential of tar. Non-proprietary preparations include crude coal-tar, which should be used under hospital supervision. It is a high-temperature, unrefined distillate diluted in white soft paraffin 1–5%. Occasionally, higher concentrations are used, but this does not confer any additional therapeutic advantage. Coal-tar solution (liquor picis carbonis) may be combined with other products, such as salicylic acid, zinc oxide or corticosteroids. Proprietary refined coal-tar products of variable, undefined composition are available as bath products, an emollient base or combined with corticosteroids.

Mode of action. The therapeutically active component(s) of coal-tar and their mechanism(s) of action are poorly defined. Coal-tar may suppress DNA synthesis and thereby reduce the epidermal hyperproliferation associated with psoriasis. Tars also have photodynamic activity in the UVA and visible spectrum, but the clinical relevance of this is uncertain.

Efficacy. Coal-tar products have been used widely in dermatology for many years. Few studies have formally evaluated the efficacy of these products, and interpretation of any results is complicated by their highly variable composition.

Use of a coal-tar 5% solution has been shown to produce a 48% mean improvement in disease severity, compared with 35% using emollients alone. Coal-tar 15% solution in aqueous cream is less effective, and also less irritating, than calcipotriol. Coal-tar 1% cream is probably as effective as a mild steroid.

In practice, coal-tar is rarely used alone. In an outpatient setting, coal-tar solution (5–15%) in combination with a topical corticosteroid, such as betamethasone valerate (0.025%), is a useful topical preparation for chronic plaque psoriasis. However, there are no studies demonstrating any superior efficacy over corticosteroid alone. Under hospital supervision, crude coal-tar distillates, used in a similar manner to dithranol (see pages 44–45), can be extremely effective for extensive chronic plaque psoriasis and may be used in situations where dithranol is contraindicated, such as poorly defined or very small plaque disease. Similarly, persistent acral psoriasis (on the hands and feet) may respond to crude coal-tar or coal-tar soaks. Use of these forms of therapy requires significant patient motivation and time, and supervision by a trained dermatological nurse.

Coal-tar is also widely used in combination with phototherapy (see page 52). For example, Goekerman's regimen combines daily coal-tar baths, applications under occlusion and UVB. In hospital or day-care settings this may produce long remissions.

Side effects, safety and cosmetic acceptability. Coal-tar products have a distinctive smell, which some patients find unpleasant, and poor cosmetic acceptability. Staining of skin and clothing precludes use of crude coal-tar at home. Local skin irritation and, rarely, allergic contact dermatitis cause problems in some patients. Coal-tar folliculitis, particularly on the lower legs, is a well recognized side effect of crude coal-tar preparations and occlusive ointment-based products. Application in the same direction as hair growth and using tar in cream or gel bases may minimize the problem. In addition, tar should not be applied immediately before sun exposure.

Occupational exposure to coal-tar is associated with an increase in the risk of skin and uroepithelial cancer. Polycyclic aromatic hydrocarbons (carcinogens known to be present in coal-tar) have been detected in the urine of patients using coal-tar shampoos, renewing concern about the oncogenic risks of coal-tar. To date, long-term studies of psoriasis patients treated with coal-tar products have not shown an increased incidence of cancer. However, further careful epidemiological studies that take into account the confounding effects of other therapeutic modalities such as phototherapy are needed to exclude the possibility of a perhaps 2–3-fold increase in cancer risk.

Dithranol (anthralin) is a highly effective treatment with no significant long-term, local, systemic or teratogenic effects. In the UK, it has been widely and successfully used for over 80 years, but has never gained similar popularity in the USA, probably because of associated skin irritation and staining.

Non-proprietary preparations include dithranol in zinc oxide (Lassar's) paste 0.1–6% and combinations with other products, such as corticosteroids. Proprietary preparations suitable for home use are also available.

Mode of action. Dithranol inhibits DNA synthesis and cellular enzymes, in particular those involved in nucleic acid metabolism and oxidative phosphorylation. These actions may reduce the epidermal hyperproliferation seen in psoriasis.

Efficacy. Dithranol is extremely effective in psoriasis. Associated irritation and staining of perilesional skin can be minimized by applying dithranol (0.1–6%) in a non-smudging paste to affected skin only, then covering with powder and/or a stockinette to reduce smearing onto normal skin. This is left in place for up to 24 hours. The application can be reduced to 1 hour, known as short-contact dithranol, further reducing staining and burning with little change in efficacy. Because of the difficulty of application, it is usual for treatment to be given under hospital supervision or by trained dermatology nurses in specialized outpatient centers. Dithranol is frequently combined with suberythema UVB in Ingram's regimen.

The majority of patients with plaque psoriasis achieve significant disease clearance after a treatment period of 20 days, with a relapse rate of 10% per month.

Side effects, safety and cosmetic acceptability. When applied to normal skin, dithranol produces redness and symptomatic burning that reaches maximum intensity after 48–72 hours and then subsides. These effects are dose-related, so therapy should be initiated at very low concentrations. Inadvertent contact with facial skin, flexural sites and eyes can produce unpleasant burns. Brown/purple staining of skin (temporary), fabrics and furniture (permanent) is primarily due to oxidation of dithranol and further reduces cosmetic acceptability. No significant long-term toxicity has been identified.

In the UK, Dithrocream® and Micanol® have been developed for home use, but are still associated with skin burning and staining. The poor tolerability means that a high degree of patient motivation is required for treatment to be successful. Formal comparison with non-proprietary preparations has not been made.

Tazarotene is available in a gel formulation (0.05% or 0.1%).

Mode of action. Licensed in the UK and USA in 1998, tazarotene was the first topical retinoid to become available for the treatment of mild-to-moderate plaque psoriasis affecting less than 20% of the body surface area. Following application, it is rapidly metabolized to the active drug, tazarotenic acid, which, by inducing tazarotene-specific gene expression, appears to normalize the rate of epidermal keratinocyte proliferation and the differentiation of epidermal cells.

Efficacy. Compared with placebo, both the 0.05% and 0.1% preparations produce a significant improvement in scaling, plaque elevation and global severity scores in mild-to-moderate plaque psoriasis; there is little difference between the two preparations. Tazarotene has the advantage of requiring only once-daily application. Few studies have compared tazarotene with other topical therapies. In terms of overall treatment success, both concentrations of tazarotene gel have similar efficacy to twice-daily fluocinonide (0.05%) cream, a potent topical corticosteroid, following 12 weeks' therapy. Predictably, patients treated with the topical corticosteroid relapsed quickly after cessation of therapy, whereas the therapeutic benefit of tazarotene was sustained during the 12-week follow-up period. The drop-out rate for patients using tazarotene was higher than for those using the corticosteroid. Combining tazarotene with a topical corticosteroid enhances speed of response and overall efficacy, and also reduces retinoid-induced skin irritation.

Side effects, safety and cosmetic acceptability. The gel is odorless and colorless. Mild-to-moderate skin irritation occurs with both

0.05% and 0.1% preparations in 10–20% of patients. Symptoms, which generally occur within the first few weeks of therapy, include burning, redness, itching and scaling. Thus, it is important to use moisturizers either before application of tazarotene or after bathing. For the same reasons, use on inflamed or pustular psoriasis and on the face or flexural sites should be avoided.

Tazarotenic acid is detectable in the plasma of up to 69% of patients using the gel topically, and has a plasma elimination half-life of 18 hours. Tazarotene should be applied to no more than 20% of the body surface area and, in view of the potential teratogenic effects of all retinoids, must be avoided during pregnancy and lactation.

Other forms of psoriasis

Guttate psoriasis. Emollients, topical corticosteroids in combination with coal-tar solution (0.025% betamethasone valerate with 5% coal-tar solution) and vitamin D_3 analogs are all of potential value and may expedite resolution. Irritant preparations such as dithranol and tazarotene are unsuitable because the size and multiplicity of lesions makes accurate application difficult. Patients who are slow to respond to therapy will often benefit from the addition of suberythema UVB (see page 51).

Chronic palmar–plantar pustulosis does not respond to the topical therapies used in routine management of chronic plaque psoriasis. However, very potent corticosteroids, with or without occlusion, are effective. Despite the thickness of the epidermis on the palms and soles, corticosteroid-induced cutaneous atrophy remains a hazard because of the chronicity and relative treatment resistance of the disease at these sites. Combining tazarotene with corticosteroids reduces this atrophy and produces more sustained results. Patients must remain under very close supervision throughout therapy.

Pustular and erythrodermic psoriasis. Both these forms represent extremely unstable and potentially life-threatening diseases. Bland emollients and the occasional use of topical corticosteroids with mild-to-moderate potency are indicated under hospital supervision only.

Special sites

Scalp and other hairy areas. The clinical manifestations of scalp psoriasis are highly variable, ranging from mild scaling and erythema to massive hyperkeratosis and so-called 'tinea amiantacea' (Figure 4.3). Choice of topical therapy needs to be tailored to the individual's needs and may vary at different times depending on disease activity. Cosmetic acceptability of the preparation is particularly important on the scalp and face. Lotions and gels designed specifically for use on hairy areas improve ease of application onto the scalp itself, though many are alcohol-based and therefore unsuitable for use on broken skin. For severe scalp psoriasis, therapeutic efficacy can be improved significantly if someone else – either a dermatology nurse or trained relative or friend – applies the topical therapy.

Mild-to-moderate scalp psoriasis. Coal-tar shampoos, with or without a keratolytic agent such as salicylic acid, and ketoconazole shampoos are particularly useful in sebo-psoriasis. However, they can be of benefit in all forms of scalp psoriasis and may be all that is required to treat mild disease. Leaving the shampoo on for 10 minutes before rinsing may enhance efficacy.

Corticosteroids (potent or very potent, groups I–V), with or without a keratolytic agent such as salicylic acid, and calcipotriol are available as lotions or gels. Formal comparison of calcipotriol

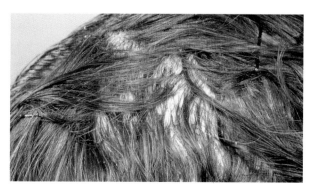

Figure 4.3 Massive hyperkeratosis (tinea amiantacea) should be gently removed with keratolytics and emollients to allow penetration of topical anti-inflammatory agents.

and the potent corticosteroid betamethasone valerate suggests that the latter is more effective. When using potent and very potent corticosteroid preparations on the scalp, particular care needs to be taken to avoid inadvertent application to the face.

Severe scalp psoriasis. Thick, adherent scale should be removed gently to allow penetration of topical anti-inflammatory agents. Suitable products contain greasy emollients, such as liquid paraffin or coconut oil, together with a keratolytic agent, such as salicylic acid, and are available in a variety of non-proprietary and proprietary preparations. They are unpleasant to use and need to be applied for at least an hour or overnight before removing with shampoo. Occasionally, dithranol is used to treat resistant scalp psoriasis, though fair or grey hair will become permanently stained.

Flexural sites, the face and genitalia are particularly vulnerable to the local side effects of corticosteroids and irritant products. Therefore, moderate potency or stronger corticosteroids, tazarotene, calcipotriol, crude or high-concentration coal-tar and dithranol are unsuitable. Creams should be used rather than ointments.

Facial psoriasis. A mild corticosteroid, with or without coal-tar solution (1%), and with or without a topical agent active against *Pityrosporum* yeasts, such as ketoconazole or co-trimoxazole, may be used, particularly in cases of sebo-psoriasis. Calcitriol or tacalcitol may also be effective. Furthermore, several uncontrolled studies suggest that tacrolimus and pimecrolimus, the new topical immunomodulator drugs licensed for use in atopic eczema, may be useful as an alternative to topical corticosteroids for facial psoriasis. Use for this indication is unlicensed. Side effects include burning and stinging.

Flexural sites (inverse psoriasis). In contrast to psoriasis in general, flexural sites frequently become secondarily infected with bacteria, usually Gram-negative organisms, and *Candida*. If necessary, a mild-to-moderate potency corticosteroid may be combined with appropriate topical antimicrobial agents, for short periods only. Again, topical tacrolimus or pimecrolimus may be useful as an alternative to topical corticosteroids. Weak antiseptic soaks (potassium permanganate or equivalent) may be added for highly exudative disease.

Ears and ear canal. The external auditory meatus and canal may become blocked with retained scale, moisture and secondary infection. The patient should be advised how to keep the ear canal as dry as possible while avoiding excessive trauma to the skin and the risk of Koebner phenomenon (see page 21). Mild-to-moderate corticosteroids combined with topical antimicrobial agents may be given as eardrops, if necessary. The presence of aggravating contact allergens should be considered in persistent disease, particularly in patients using long-term antimicrobial agents. For severe disease with pain and deafness, referral to a hospital ear, nose and throat department for ear toileting should be considered.

Nails. Nail psoriasis is difficult to manage. Topical agents are of very limited benefit and systemic therapy is rarely justified for nail disease alone. General measures include avoiding trauma and irritants, keeping nails short and the cosmetic concealment of pits and discoloration with nail gel and/or lacquer. The presence of secondary infecting agents, including *Pseudomonas*, *Candida* or dermatophytes, should be considered.

Topical therapy. Very potent corticosteroids may be rubbed into the nail fold, but duration of therapy is limited by skin atrophy. Calcipotriol can be used under occlusion but is of limited benefit. Topical tazarotene has been shown to be helpful, with or without occlusion.

Local injection of a corticosteroid, such as triamcinolone acetonide (10 mg/mL), may be given around the nail matrix and nail bed, though repeated treatments are necessary and obviously painful. These injections should be performed only by those experienced with the technique, to reduce the risk of atrophy. Subungual hyperkeratosis, nail-plate thickening and ridging will improve in the majority of patients. Onycholysis and pitting are less responsive and are often of most concern to the patient.

Systemic therapy. Improvement in nail psoriasis may occur with photochemotherapy (PUVA), methotrexate, ciclosporin or biological therapy. Acitretin may reduce subungual hyperkeratosis, though retinoid-associated thinning of the nail plate may worsen pitting and onycholysis (see Chapter 6 for further information).

Key points – topical therapy

- Approximately 70% of patients (those with mild or moderate disease) can be managed using topical therapy alone.
- Time spent detailing the practicalities of topical therapy is crucial to achieving a successful therapeutic outcome.
- A wide variety of topical therapies is available; topical corticosteroids and vitamin D_3 analogs are considered first-line therapy for most patients.
- Efficacy and cosmetic acceptability are key determinants of patient concordance with therapy.
- Consideration should be given to the body site being treated, since this influences which active ingredient and formulation should be prescribed.

Key references

Ashton RE, Andre P, Lowe NJ, Whitefield M. Anthralin: historical and current perspectives. *J Am Acad Dermatol* 1983;9:173–92.

Berth-Jones J. The emergence of vitamin D as first-line treatment for psoriasis. *J Dermatol Treatment* 1998;9:S13–18.

Larko O. Problem sites: scalp, palm and sole, nail. *Dermatol Clin* 1995;13:771–7.

Mason J, Mason AR, Cork MJ. Topical preparations for the treatment of psoriasis: a systematic review. *Br J Dermatol* 2002;146: 351–64.

Tazarotene – a topical retinoid for psoriasis. *Drug Ther Bull* 1999;37: 47–8.

Phototherapy

The beneficial effects of natural sunlight on psoriasis are well documented. Phototherapy involves whole-body exposure to artificial sources of UV radiation and is being widely and increasingly used for the treatment of extensive psoriasis resistant to topical therapy. Natural UV radiation is subdivided into UVC (below 280 nm), which is screened from the Earth's surface by ozone, UVB (280–320 nm) and UVA (320–400 nm) radiation. UVB radiation is absorbed mainly by the epidermis and is an effective treatment for psoriasis, whereas UVA penetrates the deeper layers of the dermis and is largely ineffective in psoriasis unless given in combination with a photosensitizer (see page 54).

Administration. Two sources of UV radiation are used to administer UVB phototherapy: conventional broad-band UVB (emission spectrum 270–350 nm) and the newer more effective but less widely available narrow-band UVB via the Phillips TL-01 lamp (emission spectrum 311–313 nm). Treatment must be given under the close supervision of trained staff, such as dermatology nurses or physiotherapists. The dosage schedule varies according to the patient's skin type and is based on the minimal erythema dose (MED), which is the amount of radiation required to produce faint, but definite, erythema. A meticulous record of the total cumulative UV dose for each patient is kept to avoid excessive exposure.

Indications include extensive chronic plaque psoriasis or sebo-psoriasis that is not responding adequately to topical therapy, and persistent guttate psoriasis.

Efficacy. To achieve clearance, patients receive treatment two or three times a week for 3–10 weeks, depending on disease response. Duration of disease control or remission may be prolonged by maintenance therapy, but the risks of cumulative UVB exposure must be balanced against any perceived benefits. Narrow-band UVB achieves significantly better results than broad-band UVB, probably approaching the same level of efficacy as PUVA.

The efficacy of UVB can be improved and the number of treatments can often be reduced by combining it with coal-tar, calcipotriol or tazarotene therapy. In clinical practice, UVB phototherapy is also frequently used in conjunction with dithranol, although there is no objective evidence to demonstrate superior efficacy over UVB phototherapy alone.

Concurrent use of topical corticosteroids may increase relapse rates. Systemic retinoids, such as acitretin, are widely used with PUVA and may be combined with UVB phototherapy to reduce total UVB exposure. However, initial studies of acitretin given with narrow-band UVB suggest that relapse rates may be higher than with phototherapy alone.

Side effects, safety and acceptability. In general, phototherapy is very well tolerated and is viewed by patients as an escape from the problems of topical agents. Phototherapy is well tolerated during pregnancy and can also be used in older children, though there is concern about the carcinogenic potential of administering UVB in childhood. Elderly patients may not tolerate standing in the warm, enclosed environment of the phototherapy cabinet for prolonged exposure times.

Short-term risks. Most dosage protocols aim to provide suberythema UVB to minimize short- and long-term toxicity. However, mild erythema is common and may in fact improve clearance rates. Acute sunburn can be avoided with careful dosimetry. Narrow-band UVB may be less likely to produce burning than broad-band UVB, though both are probably associated with a long-term risk of skin cancer. Xerosis (dry skin) and consequent itching usually respond to simple emollients. Rarely, photosensitive rashes such as polymorphic light eruption, lupus erythematosus and photosensitive psoriasis may be precipitated in vulnerable individuals.

Long-term risks. As with any form of chronic UV exposure, it is likely that phototherapy carries an increased risk of non-melanoma skin cancers, which increases with cumulative exposure. Broad-band UVB is probably associated with a small increase in the risk of squamous cell carcinomas, particularly in patients receiving high-level exposure (more than 300 treatments). Narrow-band UVB phototherapy has not been in clinical use for long enough to determine the associated risk precisely. On the basis of cancer-risk calculations from mouse models and efficacy data, it seems likely that the risk is at least as great as that associated with broad-band UVB, but probably less than that associated with PUVA. In view of this, phototherapy may be relatively contraindicated for patients with pre-existing risk factors for skin cancer, such as individuals who work outside, those who have already had significant amounts of phototherapy, patients with very fair skin, and those with multiple melanocytic or atypical nevi.

Home phototherapy

Although phototherapy is a popular and effective treatment for psoriasis, some patients find the repeated journeys to hospital for treatment inconvenient and expensive. Up to 50% of patients self-treat using sunbeds, either by buying a UV radiation source for use at home or attending commercial sunbed parlors.

To achieve optimal therapeutic efficacy and minimize the attendant risks of over-exposure, home use of broad-band UVB requires significant training of the patient and close supervision from a hospital base. Unnecessary continued exposure, for example for cosmetic purposes, and poor documentation of cumulative exposure are further problems, although these may be overcome by programming machines to deliver finite amounts of UV radiation. Sources sold for home use and those used in sunbed parlors tend to emit principally UVA, with little or no UVB, and therefore may be less likely to cause burning. However, compared with broad-band UVB, the therapeutic benefit of UVA is small. Thus, although home phototherapy is widely used and available, most dermatologists tend to discourage it because it is not as effective and is potentially more dangerous than hospital treatment.

Photochemotherapy (PUVA)

The use of a photosensitizing drug, methoxsalen, in combination with long-wave UVA was first reported in 1974 and has become routine therapy for the management of moderate-to-severe psoriasis. It is essential that the primary care physician, hospital staff and specialist nurses work together with the dermatologist to develop a treatment plan, both for initial clearance and maintenance therapy.

Administration. Ingestion of photosensitizing methoxsalen is followed 75 minutes later by a measured dose of UVA in a specially constructed cabinet (Figure 5.1). This combination is fraught with potential for burns, particularly when administered by inexperienced medical and nursing personnel.

The dose of methoxsalen is based on the patient's weight; the most effective dose is 0.3–0.4 mg/kg. The initial dose of UVA can

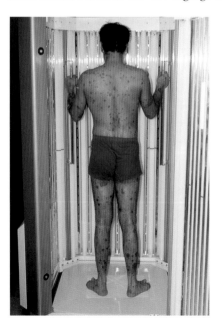

Figure 5.1 A photochemotherapy cabinet commonly used for patients with moderate-to-severe psoriasis. Bulbs emit light of specific wavelengths – UVB (broad or narrow band) or UVA.

be increased by 0.5–1 J/cm^2 at every second treatment, or until a minor degree of erythema is achieved with each treatment. It is essential that the dosage of UVA and, if necessary, oral methoxsalen, is adjusted depending on the individual patient's sensitivity and skin type. Patients with skin type I (always burns, never tans) require lower doses than patients with types V or VI (moderately or heavily pigmented skin).

Patients are usually treated twice a week. If nausea and vomiting or ocular problems develop secondary to ingestion of the sensitizing drug, or patients do not like wearing ocular protection, PUVA may be administered during bathing. The patient soaks in water containing measured amounts of the sensitizing drug before UVA exposure.

Indications. PUVA is indicated for patients with psoriasis resistant to topical therapies or with moderate-to-severe psoriasis affecting more than 10% of the body surface area. PUVA may also be beneficial for more localized, recalcitrant disease (e.g. palmar–plantar psoriasis), often in combination with retinoids. Caution must be used in patients with inflammatory psoriasis.

Contraindications. PUVA is contraindicated for patients who:
- have a history of skin cancer, particularly malignant melanoma
- are immunosuppressed
- have severe hepatic, renal or cardiovascular disease, which would preclude standing in the warm environment of the UVA unit for long periods of time
- have photosensitive diseases such as lupus erythematosus or porphyria
- are under 16 years of age.

Before starting PUVA, a full-body skin examination must be performed to rule out pre-existing premalignant or malignant skin lesions and multiple atypical nevi.

Efficacy. PUVA is extremely effective in most cases, and especially in patients with chronic, stable, plaque forms of psoriasis involving the trunk and limbs. For more verrucous or hypertrophic plaques, combination with systemic retinoids produces a more rapid effect. Remission rates with PUVA are superior to almost all other forms of therapy, including systemic treatments.

Side effects, safety and acceptability

Short-term risks. Toxicity can be a problem with the ingestion of photosensitizing agents.

Nausea and vomiting secondary to the ingestion of the sensitizing drug occurs in 10–20% of patients. However, it appears to occur less frequently with the newer form, 5-methoxypsoralen, than with the older 8-methoxypsoralen. Such effects may be reduced by taking the medication on a full stomach, or even by dividing the dose into two portions taken 30 minutes apart. Anecdotal reports suggest that consuming ginger simultaneously with methoxsalen may be beneficial. If nausea persists, antiemetics may need to be taken before ingestion of the sensitizing drug.

Pruritus is often seen after the first two or three treatments, and may be reduced by adjusting the dose of both the drug and UVA. Adequate use of emollients after and between phototherapy treatments will also help to reduce the inevitable drying effect. Itching may be aggravated by mild erythema or phototoxic reactions following each treatment.

Phototoxic reactions can be avoided by careful dosing, but are not uncommon even in patients treated by experienced personnel. The development of even slight erythema or 'sunburn' reactions should trigger a reduction in subsequent doses, or even a treatment break before resuming therapy.

Blistering is less common, appears within 24 hours of UVA exposure and peaks at 48–72 hours, with slow resolution over 3–5 days. It can be treated with wet compresses, emollients and antihistamines.

Eye protection. Psoralens remain in the eye for up to 12 hours after ingestion, so appropriate eye protection during and after treatment is critical. Current recommendations for all patients receiving oral PUVA therapy include wearing photoprotective UVA-screening glasses for 24 hours following treatment. These should be worn not only for outdoor activities, but also while driving or sitting close to a window, because UVA penetrates normal window glass. Fortunately, retrospective surveys have not shown an increased risk of posterior subcapsular cataracts in patients receiving extensive PUVA, provided such safety precautions have been taken.

Long-term risks of PUVA are significant.

Premature aging of the skin, together with thinning and bruising, occurs in patients with light skin (types I or II) who have received high-dose PUVA (multiple courses over years of therapy). In addition, an increased number of freckles (lentigines) are seen on the buttocks, hips and legs, areas not normally associated with freckling. The amount of freckling usually correlates with the number of treatments.

Skin cancer. Premalignant lesions (actinic keratoses) have been noted in increased numbers in patients with skin types I and II.

Patients who have received large cumulative doses of PUVA (in excess of 2000 J/cm^2 or more than 260 treatments) are at greater risk of squamous cell carcinoma, particularly if they are fair-skinned. There is a smaller increase in the incidence of basal cell carcinoma. The majority of PUVA-associated squamous cell carcinomas are non-invasive, though cases with metastases have been reported. In addition, an increased incidence of malignant melanoma has been reported in a special cohort of 1370 patients followed over 20 years by numerous centers in the USA. These findings have not been confirmed in Europe, however.

To reduce the overall risk of skin cancer, PUVA is frequently combined with systemic retinoids or topical therapy, such as vitamin D$_3$ and vitamin A derivatives, so that fewer treatments are needed and the cumulative UVA dose is reduced. As with phototherapy, photochemotherapy is relatively contraindicated in patients who already have risk factors for skin cancer. It should therefore be prescribed for these patients only with extreme caution.

Monitoring the UVA cabinet. The output of the fluorescent bulbs used in PUVA cabinets should be monitored carefully. A British Phototherapy Group recommendation, which can also be applied to practice in the USA, states that PUVA units should be calibrated on an annual basis by qualified medical physics department personnel. In addition, the output of the lamps should be checked, using a specific UVA-metering device, on a regular basis by medical personnel.

Patient safety. During UVA exposure, the patient should wear underwear to protect the genitals. Within the treatment room, there should be handrails and non-skid flooring, with sufficient air circulation to cool the unit. It is essential that a cut-off cord/switch

---

Key points – phototherapy and photochemotherapy

- Phototherapy (broad-band UVB and narrow-band UVB [TLO1]) is widely used for extensive chronic plaque psoriasis and sebo-psoriasis, and persistent guttate psoriasis.
- Burning and, rarely, photosensitive rashes complicate phototherapy in the short term.
- There is a small increase in the risk of non-melanoma skin cancer with long-term phototherapy.
- Photochemotherapy (PUVA) is indicated for patients with moderate-to-severe psoriasis involving more than 10% of the body surface area, and those whose psoriasis does not respond to topical therapy.
- Short-term risks of PUVA include nausea (following oral ingestion of psoralen), itching and phototoxic reactions.
- Long-term risks of PUVA include premature skin aging and skin cancer (non-melanoma and melanoma).
- In patients who already have risk factors for skin cancer, phototherapy and photochemotherapy should be prescribed only with extreme caution.

is present within the unit in case of medical emergency, and that shielding devices are in place in case of lamp breakage. A nurse should be in close attendance and should operate a hand-held timer in case the automatic timing device/computer within the UVA unit malfunctions.

After each treatment, sun exposure should be avoided for 24 hours and appropriate eye protection worn. All patients should receive regular, twice-yearly, total-body skin examinations to check for occult malignancies.

Staff protection. Protective eye wear and clothing is essential for all staff within the vicinity of the PUVA unit.

Key references

Drake LA, Ceilly RI, Dorner E et al. Guidelines of care for phototherapy and photochemotherapy. *J Am Acad Dermatol* 1994;31:643–8.

Nguyen T, Young S, Menter A. Ultraviolet B phototherapy for psoriasis. *Dermatol Ther* 1997;4:11–23.

Stern RS, Nichols KT, Vakeva LH. Malignant melanoma in patients treated for psoriasis with methoxsalen (psoralen) and ultraviolet A radiation (PUVA). *N Engl J Med* 1997;336:1041–5.

Zanoli M. Phototherapy treatment of psoriasis today. *J Am Acad Dermatol* 2003;49:578–86.

There are several important factors to consider before starting systemic therapy (Table 6.1).

To ensure appropriate safety and maximal efficacy, it is essential that a coordinated approach is adopted by the dermatologist, primary care physician, hospital staff and specialist dermatological nurse. Patient education is also important before embarking on any form of systemic therapy, particularly as all available treatments are associated with significant short- and long-term side

TABLE 6.1

Reasons to consider systemic therapy

- Poor or no response to:
  - topical therapy
  - UVB phototherapy
  - photochemotherapy (PUVA)
- Received maximum safe cumulative UV dose
- Psoriasis covers more than 10–15% of the body surface area (1% is palm-sized)
- Severe inflammatory forms of psoriasis
  - generalized pustular psoriasis
  - erythrodermic psoriasis
- Physical restrictions
  - incapacitating hand or foot psoriasis
  - associated psoriatic joint disease
  - psoriasis precluding gainful employment
- Negative impact on quality of life
  - social and personal interactions
  - severe emotional distress

effects. The benefits of disease clearance or improvement must be balanced against the risk of these side effects.

Various agents are used in the systemic treatment of psoriasis (Table 6.2). With the exception of retinoids, all are associated with varying degrees of immunosuppression. Certain groups of patients (e.g. those with cancer or those who are HIV positive) may be especially vulnerable to this aspect of treatment. Therefore, the risks of systemic therapy need to be carefully considered. Many patients in the USA are routinely assessed for HIV status before systemic therapy, including biological response modifiers (see Chapter 8). This is not the case in the UK, but patients are provided with information leaflets which indicate that those at risk of HIV infection should inform the prescribing doctor.

Methotrexate

Methotrexate has been used to treat psoriasis for over 40 years and remains the 'gold standard'. Accepted guidelines for methotrexate use have evolved in both the UK and the USA during this time.

Before starting methotrexate therapy, it is essential that patients have:
- a general physical examination
- standard laboratory blood chemistry tests
- a complete blood count
- hepatitis B and C serologies
- renal function tests
- a chest radiograph, if one has not been obtained within the previous year.

When the decision has been taken to initiate therapy and baseline studies have been completed, a single 5 mg test dose of methotrexate is given. This is a precaution to reduce the risk (albeit very small) of idiosyncratic bone-marrow suppression. A complete blood count, including a platelet count, is repeated 5–7 days after the test dose. If the result is satisfactory, the initial dose regimen for methotrexate is 10–15 mg/week. In the USA, this is usually given as either three divided doses 12 hours apart or a single dose. In the

TABLE 6.2

Drugs used in the systemic treatment of psoriasis

- Methotrexate
- Retinoids
  - etretinate
  - acitretin
- Ciclosporin
- Hydroxycarbamide*
- 6-tioguanine†
- Biological response modifiers
- Drugs affecting T-cell function
  - azathioprine
  - 6-mercaptopurine
  - mycophenolate mofetil
  - other ciclosporin-like drugs, such as tacrolimus (FK506), pimecrolimus, ascomycin and rapamycin (under evaluation)

*Hydroxycarbamide is the recommended international non-proprietary name for hydroxyurea.
†6-tioguanine is the recommended international non-proprietary name for 6-thioguanine.

UK, methotrexate is nearly always given as a single weekly dose. If it proves necessary to split the dose (e.g. because of nausea), patients in the UK receive two divided doses 12 hours apart. Methotrexate is administered orally, intramuscularly or subcutaneously. Folic acid (1 mg/day) may be given concurrently to reduce side effects such as gastric intolerance and mouth ulcers.

Laboratory evaluations are repeated every month for up to 3 months or until blood tests remain stable. Thereafter, they are repeated every 2–3 months.

In the majority of patients, an initial improvement is noted after 4 weeks of therapy, with continued gradual improvement over the next 8–12 weeks. The dose of methotrexate can be adjusted upwards, depending on response; doses of more than 25 mg/week are seldom necessary.

When adequate clearing (75–80%) has been achieved, the dose is reduced slowly by 2.5 mg/month. It is important not to discontinue methotrexate therapy abruptly because of the likelihood of destabilizing the psoriasis, which can lead to severe erythrodermic flares. Most patients will require small doses (e.g. 7.5 mg/week) for continued control. Rotation with other therapies may improve long-term remissions and reduce the need for liver biopsy, which is currently recommended after approximately 1.5 g (2–3 years) of continuous methotrexate treatment.

Contraindications. Methotrexate is contraindicated in patients who:
- are considering conception, because this drug is a teratogen (men and women should be counseled to avoid conception for at least 3 months after discontinuation of their methotrexate therapy)
- are pregnant or breastfeeding
- have a history of abnormal liver function tests, hepatitis, HIV infection or other infectious diseases (e.g. pyelonephritis or tuberculosis) or blood dyscrasias
- have an underlying malignancy
- are non-compliant or unreliable (e.g. ignoring advice to avoid alcohol).

Drug interactions. In addition to general counseling and instructions to avoid alcohol, it is important to inform patients of possible drug interactions. This includes interactions with:
- sulfonamides
- barbiturates
- trimethoprim
- non-steroidal anti-inflammatory drugs (NSAIDs)
- probenecid.

Side effects, such as fatigue, nausea and vomiting, are usually seen within 4–48 hours of dosing. These may be alleviated by concomitant folic acid use, but frequently an antiemetic is required.

There is an increased risk of bone-marrow toxicity and hepatotoxicity with high cumulative doses of methotrexate, so doses must be monitored carefully. A total cumulative dose of more than 4 g may increase the risk of liver toxicity and cirrhosis. Current guidelines recommend a liver biopsy after approximately 1.5 g (2–3 years) of continuous methotrexate treatment. Recently, however, measurement of type III serum procollagen has been adopted by some centers in the UK and the USA as a non-invasive marker of hepatic fibrosis, which has reduced the need for 'routine' liver biopsy.

The rotational approach to management, in which there is a 'drug holiday' of 1–2 years 'off' methotrexate, with less than a total of 1.5 g of the drug being administered during each course 'on', may also reduce the need for liver biopsies.

Another less frequently noted side effect is methotrexate-induced pneumonitis. Patients should be instructed to report any persistent, non-productive, dry cough; appropriate evaluation and radiography should be carried out if such a cough develops.

Systemic retinoids

The first systemic retinoid used to treat psoriasis was etretinate, which was introduced approximately 20 years ago. It has recently been superseded by its natural metabolite, acitretin. The usual dose regimen for acitretin is 25 mg/day or 0.25–0.5 mg/kg/day. As with methotrexate therapy, when a reasonable improvement has been achieved, the dose can be reduced slowly.

Combination of a systemic retinoid with either UVB or PUVA treatment has the advantage that both the dose of the systemic retinoid and the number of phototherapy treatments can be reduced. Systemic retinoids may also be combined or overlapped with other systemic agents, such as ciclosporin or hydroxycarbamide (see Chapter 7).

Contraindications. Systemic retinoids are major teratogens and are therefore contraindicated in women of childbearing age. Following cessation of acitretin therapy, women are advised to avoid conception for a minimum of 3 years in the USA and 2 years in the UK.

Side effects. Although not as effective as methotrexate, acitretin has fewer side effects. This is particularly true regarding hepatotoxicity, with idiosyncratic retinoid hepatitis occurring less commonly. However, acitretin tends to increase serum triglycerides and, to a lesser extent, cholesterol levels. Careful management is required, including dose reduction, specific diet and, if necessary, appropriate drug therapy.

The most significant side effect is mucocutaneous toxicity. Dryness of the lips, nose, eyes, hair, skin and mucous membranes is inevitable. Many patients also complain of a sticky, clammy feel to the skin, as well as a moderate degree of reversible hair loss, which is seen more commonly in women and at higher doses.

Ciclosporin

Ciclosporin was first reported as therapy for psoriasis about 20 years ago. Awareness of the effect of this drug on T cells has stimulated research into the immunopathogenesis of psoriasis, leading to better understanding of the disease.

Approved for the treatment of psoriasis in the UK in 1993 and in the USA in 1997, ciclosporin has proved to be an excellent therapy for widespread recalcitrant psoriasis and is well tolerated by the majority of patients. It is probably best used as interventional therapy, with slow tapering of the dose once adequate control is obtained. Wherever possible, therapy should be limited to short periods of up to 1 year, with rotation to other systemic agents or phototherapy in order to avoid long-term monotherapy.

Ciclosporin is usually given in initial doses of 3–4 mg/kg/day, although the new micro-emulsion formulation may be used at slightly lower doses. In general, the more inflammatory the psoriasis, the more dramatic the response. Complete clearing of even the most generalized erythrodermic or pustular disease is possible within 3–6 weeks of beginning therapy. Less dramatic results are seen in patients with chronic plaque psoriasis, who often require 4 months of therapy for optimal improvement.

Drug interactions. Careful coordination of medication between the dermatologist and the primary care physician is essential. There is the potential for interaction with various other drugs, including certain antibiotics (e.g. erythromycin), sulfonamides and antifungals (e.g. fluconazole, itraconazole and ketoconazole). A complete list of drug interactions is available from the manufacturer.

Side effects. The most common side effects are hypertension and nephrotoxicity. Before starting therapy, full clinical, laboratory and blood pressure evaluations should be carried out to provide baseline values. It is essential to monitor blood pressure each week, because it often increases slowly from baseline before any change in renal function is noted. An increase from a baseline of 120/70 mmHg to 138/85 mmHg, for example, should alert the physician to early nephrotoxicity.

If patients remain normotensive and serum creatinine does not increase above 30% of baseline, ciclosporin may be continued effectively for a year or more. European studies have recently reported up to 10-year usage, with 50% of a small group of patients showing evidence of renal impairment, including fibrosis, on biopsy findings.

In addition to standard urinalysis and serum creatinine measurement, creatinine or glomerular clearance should be assessed if long-term therapy (more than 6 months) is likely.

Ciclosporin should be used with caution in patients who have had significant amounts of PUVA (i.e. more than 100 treatments) because of the increased risk of skin cancer. A recent prospective study of 1252 patients who were followed for 5 years found no increased incidence of non-skin malignancy when compared with the general population; however, skin cancers were substantially increased in patients who had received prior PUVA therapy.

In addition, gingival hyperplasia and increased hair growth are not infrequent side effects of ciclosporin therapy.

Hydroxycarbamide

Hydroxycarbamide (the recommended international non-proprietary name for hydroxyurea) is considered to be a second-line therapy for psoriasis, with improvement occurring more slowly than with methotrexate, systemic retinoids or ciclosporin. Some consider that it is underused in psoriasis treatment.

The majority of patients achieve clearance of approximately 50–60%. Doses of 1–2 g/day are usually required and produce an inevitable increase in mean corpuscular volume. Provided that the white cell count does not fall below 3×10^6/mL and the hemoglobin, hematocrit and platelet count are not significantly reduced, the drug may be used as long-term therapy with minimal effects on other blood chemistries.

Hydroxycarbamide may be combined with low-dose systemic retinoids and may be of value in treating the palmar–plantar form of psoriasis.

Side effects. Major systemic side effects are much less likely than with other commonly used systemic treatments. Bone-marrow suppression is the most important adverse effect.

6-tioguanine

6-tioguanine (6-thioguanine) is a purine analog antimetabolite used to treat patients with psoriasis that has been recalcitrant to other systemic therapies. It is taken orally, and several dosing strategies have been devised in an effort to minimize bone-marrow suppression. As with methotrexate, baseline laboratory values should be obtained so that they can be compared with the results of subsequent monitoring. This should include baseline measurement of the thiopurine methyltransferase (TPMT) level; a minority of patients have a low level of this enzyme and should not be treated with 6-tioguanine because of the risk of bone-marrow suppression.

One study found minimal bone-marrow suppression with an initial dose of 80 mg twice weekly. The dose can be titrated upward to gain the desired effect, using increments of 20 mg every 2–4 weeks. Maintenance doses generally range from 120 mg twice weekly to 160 mg three times per week.

Side effects. Myelosuppression is the most common adverse event associated with 6-tioguanine. Gastrointestinal side effects, including nausea, vomiting and reflux, are also common.

Biological response modifiers

The role of biological response modifiers in the treatment of psoriasis is described in Chapter 8.

Other systemic therapies

Various other drugs that affect T-cell function may be used in the treatment of severe psoriasis, including:

- azathioprine
- 6-mercaptopurine
- mycophenolate mofetil.

Other ciclosporin-like drugs, such as tacrolimus (FK506), pimecrolimus, ascomycin and rapamycin, are currently under evaluation.

Key points – systemic therapy

- Psoriasis is a systemic disease of immune system dysregulation and therefore a significant proportion (perhaps as many as one-third) of patients require systemic medication.
- Side effects of systemic therapies for psoriasis include myelosuppression, hepatotoxicity and nephrotoxicity.
- Teratogenicity limits the use of methotrexate and acitretin.

Key references

Heydendael VM, Spuls PI, Opmeer BC et al. Methotrexate versus cyclosporine in moderate-to-severe chronic plaque psoriasis. *N Engl J Med* 2003;349:658–65.

Lebwohl M. Acitretin in combination with UVB or PUVA. *J Am Acad Dermatol* 1999:41: S22–4.

Lebwohl M, Ali S. Treatment of psoriasis. Part 2. Systemic therapies. *J Am Acad Dermatol* 2001;45:649–61;662–4.

Lebwohl M, Ellis C, Gottlieb A et al. Cyclosporine consensus conference: with emphasis on the treatment of psoriasis. *J Am Acad Dermatol* 1998;39:464–75.

Lowe NJ, Wieder JM, Rosenbach A et al. Long-term low-dose cyclosporine therapy for severe psoriasis: effects on renal function and structure. *J Am Acad Dermatol* 1996;35:710–19.

McLeod HL, Siva C. The thiopurine S-methyltransferase gene locus – implications for clinical pharmacogenomics. *Pharmacogenomics* 2002;3:89–98.

Menter A, Barker JN. Psoriasis in practice. *Lancet* 1991;338:231–4.

Paul CF, Ho VC, McGeown C et al. Risk of malignancies in psoriasis patients treated with cyclosporine: a 5 y cohort study. *J Invest Dermatol* 2003;120: 211–16.

Roenigk HH Jr. Acitretin combination therapy. *J Am Acad Dermatol* 1999;41:S18–21.

Roenigk HH Jr, Auerbach R, Maibach H et al. Methotrexate in psoriasis: consensus conference. *J Am Acad Dermatol* 1998;38: 478–85.

Silvis NG, Levine N. Pulse dosing of thioguanine in recalcitrant psoriasis. *Arch Dermatol* 1999;135:433–7.

Spuls PI, Whitkamp L, Bossuyt PM, Bos JD. A systematic review of five systemic treatments for severe psoriasis: reply. *Br J Dermatol* 1998;139:757–8.

Fortunately, there is now an impressive array of treatments for all forms of psoriasis, whether mild, moderate or severe. Topical psoriasis therapy is analogous to the use of NSAIDs in rheumatoid arthritis, another immune-mediated disease. If adequate control of psoriasis is not achieved with topical therapy, the next line of treatment is UVB phototherapy and then, if necessary, PUVA, where available. If these types of treatment are inappropriate or fail, the patient is given systemic therapy. This is similar to the use of disease-modifying antirheumatic drugs in rheumatoid therapy, with UVB and PUVA being analogous to gold and 4-aminoquinoline therapy. Methotrexate and ciclosporin are used in the more severe forms of both psoriasis and rheumatoid disease.

In the UK, PUVA is increasingly being reserved for older patients, because the risk of skin cancer increases over time, and those who receive PUVA and immunosuppressants have a greatly escalated risk. Hence, systemic therapy may be used relatively early in younger patients who have severe disease.

Since psoriasis is a chronic disease, long-term therapy is required, which raises the potential problem of cumulative toxicities. Rotational, combination and sequential therapeutic strategies offer the potential advantages of reduced side effects and increased efficacy, while maintaining longer term control and reducing the frequency of inevitable relapses.

The schema outlined below is theoretical; in practice, the appropriate choice of therapy for an individual will be based on the history and physical examination, together with consideration of quality of life and family planning issues.

Rotational therapy

The initial concept of rotational therapy proposed by Weinstein in 1993 involved PUVA, methotrexate, systemic retinoids and UVB plus tar preparations, each used in cycles of approximately 1 year. Other investigators have since added other treatments to the rotation and lengthened the duration of the individual treatments.

The rationale underlying rotational therapy is to discontinue one medication as it is approaching its cumulative toxic dose and then 'rotate' to a different drug that maintains the response but has a different toxicity profile. For example, a patient could theoretically be maintained on methotrexate for several years and, as the cumulative dose neared 1.5 g, could then be rotated to another treatment. If the switch were made to a non-hepatotoxic drug such as ciclosporin, remission could be maintained and the recommended liver biopsy could possibly be avoided.

Later, as initial signs of hypertension and nephrotoxicity developed with ciclosporin, the patient could be rotated to phototherapy. This would need to be done cautiously because increased incidence of non-melanoma cutaneous malignancies has been found in patients who have been treated with both ciclosporin and phototherapy.

Other reasons to rotate therapy include side effects, loss of efficacy and onset of a new flare.

Combination therapy

Combination therapy is often required for long-term control of psoriasis, as for rheumatoid disease. It is important to recognize that even the most potent systemic agents, such as ciclosporin and methotrexate, may not achieve the therapeutic goal when used alone. Various combinations of topical, systemic and light treatment may be needed to clear localized resistant patches and reduce the need for sustained longer term systemic therapy. Several combination strategies have been described, with most achieving clinical effects at lower doses than when either drug is used alone. Commonly used systemic/phototherapy combinations include: retinoid (acitretin) + UVB; retinoid + PUVA; and methotrexate + UVB.

The combination of low-dose ciclosporin and methotrexate is approved in the UK and the USA for rheumatoid disease but has not yet been formally approved for psoriasis. However, if a patient is receiving one of these drugs, it is possible to slowly reduce the dose and cautiously add the second drug in an 'overlap approach' for a 3–4-month period. The initial drug can then be discontinued while continuing with the second. This limits the possibility of a relapse or rebound of disease, which sometimes occurs when a drug is discontinued, and helps to maintain longer term control and remissions.

The great benefit of a combined or rotational approach is longer term remissions than may have been achieved with any individual modality, as well as reductions in individual drug toxicities (e.g. hepatotoxicity with methotrexate and nephrotoxicity with ciclosporin).

Sequential therapy

The paradigm of sequential therapy was first proposed in 1999 by Koo, who suggested that certain medications could be used to clear psoriasis and others to maintain remission. Using this sequential approach, relatively toxic agents such as methotrexate can be used to achieve improvement quickly when psoriasis flares. This is followed by transition to long-term maintenance with potentially less toxic modalities such as phototherapy or acitretin.

On average, no single treatment modality, with the possible exception of PUVA and perhaps some of the biological response modifying drugs (see Chapter 8), is likely to achieve remission for more than 3 months. Withdrawal of individual therapies, with subsequent relapses and destabilization of disease, certainly has a negative impact on the person's well-being and quality of life. Therefore, it is crucial that any long-term course of therapy is planned and coordinated by the dermatologist, primary care physician and patient in order to reduce patient discontent and cumulative, long-term side effects.

Key points – rotational, combined and sequential therapies

• Psoriasis is a chronic disease requiring long-term therapy.
• All systemic medications used for psoriasis can have limiting side effects and toxicities.
• Rotational, combination and sequential therapeutic strategies can reduce side effects and increase efficacy, while maintaining longer term control of the psoriasis and reducing the frequency and severity of inevitable relapses.

Key references

Cather J, Menter A. Novel therapies for psoriasis. *Am J Clin Dermatol* 2002;3:159–73.

Koo J. Systemic sequential therapy of psoriasis: a new paradigm for improved therapeutic results. *J Am Acad Dermatol* 1999;41:S25–8.

Lebwohl M, Drake L, Menter A et al. Consensus conference: acitretin in combination with UVB or PUVA in the treatment of psoriasis. *J Am Acad Dermatol* 2001;45:544–53.

Menter A, Abramovits W. Rational, sequential and combination regimens in the treatment of psoriasis. *Dermatol Ther* 1999;11:88–95.

Menter MA, See JA, Amend WJ et al. Proceedings of the Psoriasis Combination and Rotation Therapy Conference. Deer Valley, Utah, 7–9 October 1994. *J Am Acad Dermatol* 1996;34:315–21.

Paul CF, Ho VC, McGeown C et al. Risk of malignancies in psoriasis patients treated with cyclosporine: a 5 year cohort study. *J Invest Dermatol* 2003;120: 211–16.

Weinstein GD, White GM. An approach to the treatment of moderate to severe psoriasis with rotational therapy. *J Am Acad Dermatol* 1993;28:454–9.

Laura Winterfield

As discussed in Chapter 1 (page 10), psoriasis is an immune-mediated disease characterized by infiltration of T lymphocytes into the dermis and epidermis. The driving T-cell population in psoriatic lesions is activated memory effector T cells. To reach the effector state, T cells must first be activated by antigen-presenting cells (APCs). This requires three interactions between the T cell and the APC:

- non-specific reversible binding of the T cell to the APC through interactions of surface molecules on the two cells
- recognition of the major histocompatibility complex molecule on the APC by the antigen-specific T-cell receptor
- costimulatory signal from the APC to the T cell via surface molecules, leading to production of interleukin 2 (IL-2), which binds to the IL-2 receptor on the T-cell surface; several different molecular interactions may function as costimulatory signals (Figure 8.1).

Once the T cell has been activated by the APC, it enters the bloodstream and migrates back to the skin. This migration is achieved by the lymphocyte function-associated antigen 1 (LFA1) complex on the T cell binding to an intercellular adhesion molecule 1 (ICAM1) on an endothelial cell in the cutaneous vasculature.

Initial skin activation is required for APCs to migrate from skin and interact with T cells (proinflammatory state), and, similarly, chemokines and proinflammatory cytokines are needed for T cells to enter the skin. These chemokines and cytokines are derived from endogenous skin cells (dendritic cells, macrophages, keratinocytes etc.) as well as recruited cells.

The T cells in psoriatic lesions secrete proinflammatory cytokines of the T1 type, including IL-2, interferon γ and tumor necrosis factor α (TNFα). These cytokines induce epidermal and vascular changes that lead to the clinical changes seen in psoriatic plaques.

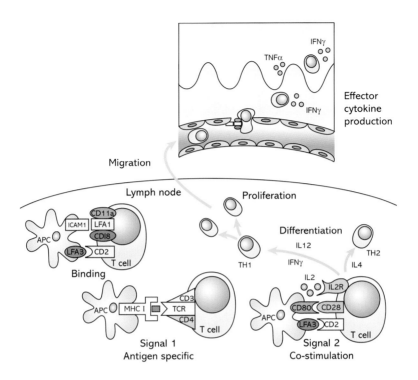

Figure 8.1 Immunopathogenesis of psoriasis. Antigen-presenting cells (APCs) migrate from the skin to the lymph node, where they encounter naïve T cells. These T cells become activated through a series of three interactions with APCs (see text). Once activated, the T cells migrate back to the skin, where they secrete proinflammatory cytokines such as interleukin 2 (IL-2) and interferon γ (IFNγ). This induces further production of proinflammatory cytokines, including tumor necrosis factor α (TNFα). ICAM, intercellular adhesion molecule; IL-2R, IL-2 receptor; LFA, lymphocyte function-associated antigen; MHC, major histocompatibility complex; TH, T-helper cell; TCR, T-cell receptor.

As specific details of the immunopathogenesis of psoriasis have been elucidated, new therapies have been developed which target the aberrant immune cells and molecules that trigger the development of psoriatic plaques. Biological response modifiers are a new class of drugs used to treat immune-mediated diseases, including psoriasis. They are designed specifically to interfere with T-cell activation and effector function in order to prevent the inflammatory effects characteristic of this group of diseases. Many of these drugs are also effective in treating psoriatic arthritis, a debilitating inflammatory arthritis that may affect up to 25% of patients with moderate-to-severe psoriatic skin disease (see Chapter 9).

Definition and background

Biological response modifiers (or 'biologics') are proteins derived from recombinant DNA technology, hybridomas, blood and whole human cells. Three main types of biologics are used to treat inflammatory diseases:
- recombinant cytokines or growth factors
- monoclonal antibodies
- fusion proteins.

These drugs are named according to their structure (Figure 8.2). Biologics are large molecules and administration is via injection or infusion; as yet, no oral biological agents are available.

Strategies to treat psoriasis

There are four major ways in which the various biologics are active against psoriasis (Table 8.1).

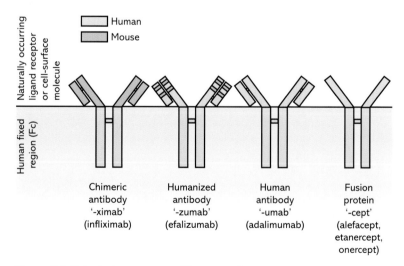

Figure 8.2 Biological response modifier nomenclature.

Elimination of pathogenic T cells. Alefacept, a fusion protein combining LFA3 with the Fc portion of human IgG, is able to eliminate pathogenic T cells. The drug binds to CD2 on T cells to block costimulation by LFA3 on APCs (see Figure 8.1).

The main side effect of alefacept is CD4 suppression, so it is essential to monitor the CD4 count weekly. If the CD4 count is higher than 250 cell/μL, the weekly dose of alefacept should be maintained. Individual courses last for 12 weeks, followed by 12 weeks without alefacept.

Blockade of T-cell activation/costimulation/migration can be achieved with efalizumab. This anti-CD11a humanized monoclonal antibody binds to CD11a, which is a component of LFA1 on T cells, thereby preventing interaction of LFA1 with ICAM1 on APCs and hence blocking the costimulatory signal.

The LFA1–ICAM1 interaction is also involved in T-cell migration into inflamed tissue; this is a second mechanism of action against psoriasis for this drug.

Alteration of T-cell proliferative signals/immune deviation can also be achieved with efalizumab.

Blocking proinflammatory effector cytokines. Four agents are known to block effector cytokines: etanercept, infliximab, adalimumab and onercept.

- Etanercept is a fusion protein composed of the human TNF receptor II plus the Fc region of human IgG1. It binds soluble and cell-surface TNFα and TNFβ.
- Infliximab is a chimeric monoclonal antibody that specifically binds soluble and surface-bound TNFα.
- Adalimumab, a monoclonal antibody with human-derived heavy and light chain variable regions and human IgG1:κ constant regions, binds TNFα.
- Onercept, a recombinant, unmodified, fully human, soluble type I TNF receptor (p55), also acts as an anti-TNF agent.

TABLE 8.1

Characteristics of biological response modifiers

Name	Strategy*	Structure	Dose regimen
Alefacept	1	Fusion protein: LFA3 with human Fc	7.5 mg i.v. or 15 mg i.m. every week for 12 weeks[†]
Efalizumab	2, 3	Humanized monoclonal anti-CD11a antibody	1 mg/kg s.c. every week
Etanercept	4	Fusion protein: soluble TNFα receptor with human Fc	50 mg s.c. twice a week for 12 weeks, then 25 mg twice a week (FDA-approved regimen)
Infliximab	4	Chimeric anti-TNFα monoclonal antibody	5 mg/kg i.v. infusion at 0, 2 and 6 weeks; then every 8 weeks
Adalimumab	4	Monoclonal anti-TNFα antibody with human-derived heavy and light chain variable regions and human IgG1 Fc constant regions	40 mg s.c. every 2 weeks
Onercept	4	Recombinant, unmodified, fully human, soluble, type I TNFα receptor (p55)	150 mg s.c. three times a week

*Strategy 1, elimination of pathogenic T cells; strategy 2, blocking T-cell activation/costimulation/migration; strategy 3, alteration of T-cell proliferative signals/immune deviation; strategy 4, blocking effector cytokines (TNFα).

[†]In the USA, only 15 mg i.m. is available.

FDA, Food and Drug Administration; i.m., intramuscularly; i.v., intravenously; LFA3, lymphocyte function-associated antigen 3; s.c., subcutaneously; TNFα, tumor necrosis factor α.

PASI data[‡] 50/75/90	Selected side effects	FDA approval/ stage of development
50/33/NA[§] at any time before study endpoint	CD4 suppression; must monitor CD4 weekly	Moderate-to-severe psoriasis
55.7/27/NA[§] after 12 weeks of therapy; 67/44/15[§] after 24 weeks of therapy	Headache, nausea, chills	Moderate-to-severe psoriasis
74/49/22[§] after 12 weeks of therapy 77/59/30[§] after 24 weeks of therapy	Injection site reactions; multiple-sclerosis-like syndrome[¶]	Moderate-to-severe psoriasis; psoriatic arthritis, rheumatoid arthritis; ankylosing spondylitis
97/88/58[§] after 10 weeks of therapy (three i.v. infusions)	Infusion reactions, reactivation of tuberculosis[¶]	Crohn's disease, rheumatoid arthritis Phase III for psoriasis began in October 2003; data not yet available
NA/57–81/NA[§] (PASI 75 is 57% with treatment every other week, 81% with treatment every week)	Injection site reactions, upper respiratory tract infections, nausea, headache (early Phase II data for psoriasis)[¶]	Rheumatoid arthritis Phase II/III for psoriasis
74/54/NA[§] after 12 weeks of therapy	Injection site reactions (early Phase II data only)	Phase II for psoriasis and psoriatic arthritis

[‡]PASI, Psoriasis Area and Severity Index, a measure of erythema, induration and scale across four major body sites; PASI 50/75/90, 50%/75%/90% improvement in the baseline PASI score.

[§]The first figure in this column is the percentage of patients achieving PASI 50, the second is the percentage achieving PASI 75 and the third is the percentage achieving PASI 90. NA, no data available.

[¶]Extensive experience has been gained with all three TNF blockers in rheumatoid arthritis and Crohn's disease.

Role of the biological response modifiers

Biological response modifiers are likely to revolutionize the treatment of moderate-to-severe psoriasis. They have the advantage over traditional therapies of no apparent organ toxicity, including renal toxicity and hepatotoxicity. Individual drugs may prove to induce sustained, drug-free remissions in patients with psoriasis.

Long-term safety data for treating psoriasis are still lacking, but hundreds of thousands of patients with Crohn's disease and rheumatoid arthritis have been treated for more than 5 years with etanercept or infliximab.

Studies are under way to determine the optimal ways of combining biological agents with traditional therapies such as phototherapy, retinoids, methotrexate and topical medication. Eventually, it may be possible to add multiple biological therapies into a combination regimen.

While the goal for patients is long-term disease-free remissions and improved quality of life, overall cost and long-term safety will be key issues in determining the significance of biological therapies for treating psoriasis.

Key points – biological response modifiers

- Biological response modifiers ('biologics') are a new class of drugs, widely available for several years, that target specific molecules involved in the immunopathogenesis of immune-mediated diseases such as psoriasis, psoriatic arthritis, rheumatoid arthritis and Crohn's disease.
- The biologics currently available or in clinical trials are all given by injection (subcutaneous, intramuscular or intravenous).
- Evidence to date suggests that biologics do not have toxic effects on internal organs.
- Some of these agents may offer long-term remissions for patients with psoriasis.
- Cost and long-term safety will be important in determining the future role of biologics in the treatment of psoriasis.

Key references

Chaudhari U, Romano P, Mulcahy LD et al. Efficacy and safety of infliximab monotherapy for plaque-type psoriasis: a randomized trial. *Lancet* 2001;357:1842–7.

Gottlieb AB, Papp KA, Lynde CW et al. Subcutaneous efalizumab (anti-CD11a) is effective in the treatment of moderate to severe plaque psoriasis: pooled results of two phase III clinical trials. Poster presented at the 60th Annual Meeting of the American Academy of Dermatology, 22–27 February 2002; New Orleans, LA.

Krueger GG, Papp KA, Sough DB et al. A randomized, double-blind, placebo-controlled phase III study evaluating efficacy and tolerability of two courses of alefacept in patients with chronic plaque psoriasis. *J Am Acad Dermatol* 2002;47:821–33.

Kupper TS. Immunologic targets in psoriasis. *N Engl J Med* 2003; 349:1987–90.

Leonardi CL, Powers JL, Matheson RT et al. Etanercept Psoriasis Study Group. Etanercept as monotherapy in patients with psoriasis. *N Engl J Med* 2003;349: 2014–22.

Mease PJ, Goffe BS, Metz J et al. Etanercept in the treatment of psoriatic arthritis and psoriasis: a randomized trial. *Lancet* 2000; 356:385–90.

Mehlis SL, Gordon KB. The immunology of psoriasis and biologic immunotherapy. *J Am Acad Dermatol* 2003;49:S44–50

Philip Mease

Psoriatic arthritis is a common autoimmune inflammatory condition affecting the joints and entheses of patients with psoriasis. Clinical manifestations are heterogeneous and vary widely in severity.

The disease is underdiagnosed and often undertreated. However, recent advances in therapy offer the prospect of more complete disease control, including the prevention of joint destruction. It is therefore important for a correct diagnosis to be reached promptly.

History and classification

An association between psoriasis and a form of inflammatory arthritis was first suggested in the 1850s. However, the characterization of psoriatic arthritis as a distinct form of arthritis was not fully articulated until the early 1960s, by Wright, Baker and others. Until that time, it was considered to be a variant of rheumatoid arthritis seen in individuals with concomitant psoriasis.

Psoriatic arthritis was formally recognized as a distinct entity by the American Rheumatism Association in 1964. Further observations about familial associations, common clinical characteristics and, ultimately, HLA associations in the early 1970s placed psoriatic arthritis in the group known as seronegative spondylarthropathies, such as ankylosing spondylitis and reactive arthritis.

In the mid 1970s, Moll and Wright, in Leeds, UK, characterized five subsets of psoriatic arthritis (Table 9.1). This classification still prevails. However, an international study is under way that aims to develop a new classification scheme, based on laboratory and radiographic findings, as well as clinical variables.

Clinical manifestations

Although psoriatic arthritis may present in adolescence, onset is most common in patients in their 20s or 30s, occurring with equal prevalence in men and women. In 75% of cases, onset of skin

TABLE 9.1

Clinical subsets of psoriatic arthritis

- Oligoarticular ($\leq$ 5 joints) – asymmetrical
- Polyarticular – may be asymmetrical or symmetrical
- Distal interphalangeal predominant
- Mutilans
- Spondylitis predominant (especially sacroiliac joint)

disease precedes the development of arthritis, often by a decade or more. In 15% of cases, the onset of skin and joint disease is simultaneous, and in only 10% do the joint manifestations precede the appearance of skin lesions.

It is especially challenging for the clinician to make an accurate diagnosis of psoriatic arthritis when joint manifestations appear before signs of skin disease. In such cases, confirmatory diagnosis may be delayed until skin lesions appear, even when there is strong suspicion based on clinical and radiographic appearance. Table 9.2 lists the disorders that should be considered in the differential diagnosis of psoriatic arthritis.

The most common variant of psoriatic arthritis, at least initially, is oligoarticular, asymmetrical arthritis (Figure 9.1). Patients with this form of the disease exhibit characteristic inflammatory changes of joint swelling, redness, pain and stiffness, involving five or fewer

TABLE 9.2

Differential diagnosis of psoriatic arthritis

- Osteoarthritis (especially given similar distal interphalangeal involvement)
- Rheumatoid arthritis (especially polyarticular variant, if symmetrical)
- Ankylosing spondylitis (if there is spondylitic involvement)
- Gout (if oligoarticular)
- Tendonitis (if there is enthesial involvement)

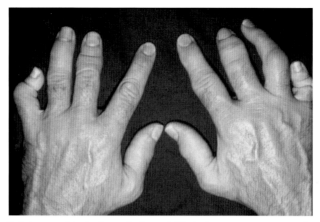

Figure 9.1 Asymmetrical, oligoarticular arthritis is the most common variant of psoriatic arthritis, at least initially. Image © 1972-2004 American College of Rheumatology Clinical Slide Collection. Used with permission.

joints. These changes may be chronic, or may wax and wane. At this stage, the disease may not be disabling unless the inflammation is severe or the joints involved are critical for activities of daily living, work or recreational function. Occasionally, the spine will be involved, with patients typically noting pain and stiffness in the lower back, sacroiliac joint areas and neck.

The patient may also complain of non-articular musculoskeletal pain and stiffness, particularly at tendon or ligament insertion sites (enthesitis) such as the heel insertions of the Achilles tendon or plantar fascia, as well as ligamentous insertion sites around the chest wall and pelvis. Dactylitis, or 'sausage digit change', appears to be a combination of joint inflammation and enthesitis in the shaft of the digit (Figure 9.2). Rarely, such non-articular involvement will be the only manifestation of psoriatic arthritis. Non-musculoskeletal inflammatory symptoms may also appear episodically, including iritis.

As the disease evolves over time, there is a tendency for more joints to be involved in a polyarticular fashion. In some patients, this will be more symmetrical in pattern, similar to rheumatoid arthritis. At this stage, it is more common for individuals to experience disability and deforming changes of the joints.

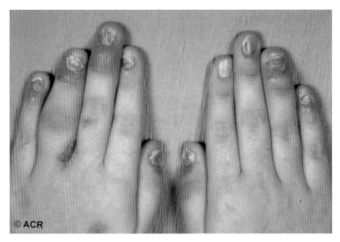

Figure 9.2 Dactylitis of the left fourth (ring) finger. There is also distal interphalangeal inflammation in the left third to fifth and right fourth and fifth fingers, together with nail changes that are characteristic of psoriasis. Image © 1972-2004 American College of Rheumatology Clinical Slide Collection. Used with permission.

Radiographic and laboratory features

In addition to the clinical features discussed above, unique radiographic features help to distinguish psoriatic arthritis. These include the so-called 'pencil-in-cup' change (Figure 9.3), periostitis, asymmetrical erosive changes and/or ankylosis, distal digit tuft resorption and proliferative new bone formation at the entheses.

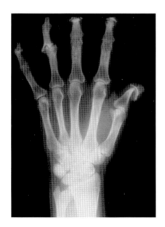

Figure 9.3 The 'pencil-in-cup' radiological deformity in a patient with psoriatic arthritis, most prominently seen in the interphalangeal joint of the first finger. Image © 1972-2004 American College of Rheumatology Clinical Slide Collection. Used with permission.

In the spine, hallmarks of psoriatic arthritis may include asymmetrical sacroiliitis and asymmetrical syndesmophytes bridging vertebral bodies.

Blood testing for rheumatoid factor is usually, although not invariably, negative. Acute phase reactants, erythrocyte sedimentation rate (ESR) and C-reactive protein (CRP) may be elevated, but there may be no correlation between these values and the degree of disease activity. In juvenile psoriatic arthritis, which is rare, tests for antinuclear antibodies may prove positive.

Explosive new onset or worsening of psoriasis and/or psoriatic arthritis may prompt HIV testing, because a higher prevalence of these diseases has been reported in patients who have AIDS.

In some patients, especially early in the disease process, all laboratory and radiographic findings may be normal. This is often frustrating for the clinician and patient alike, as diagnostic confirmation is sought.

Prevalence

Given the heterogeneous manifestations of psoriatic arthritis and the potential for incorrect diagnosis, it is not surprising that the literature offers a wide range of prevalence figures for this disease.

It is generally accepted that the prevalence of psoriasis is just over 2% in the North American and European populations. Reports of the prevalence of psoriatic arthritis among those with psoriasis have ranged from 5% to 42%. Lower percentages are suggested when a simple community survey or patient chart review is carried out. Higher percentages are derived when a more detailed prospective patient analysis is performed.

It is likely that the true prevalence is around 25%. Bearing this in mind may prompt the physician to obtain a more detailed history and conduct a more thorough physical examination for musculoskeletal problems in a patient with psoriasis.

Pathogenesis

Genetics. There is a strong familial tendency for both psoriasis and psoriatic arthritis. A variety of HLA antigens have been associated with psoriatic arthritis, including B13, B17, B27, B38, B39, Cw6, DR4 and DR7. Patients with HLA-B27 are more likely to have spine manifestations.

Immunology. As in other autoimmune inflammatory diseases, such as rheumatoid arthritis and psoriasis, there is upregulation of macrophage and T-cell activation, with a consequent outpouring of cytokines which promote the inflammatory cascade. These prominently include TNFα, IL1 and others. In contrast to rheumatoid synovium, there is less lymphoid infiltrate, more vascularity and fewer plasma cells and macrophages.

As in rheumatoid arthritis, the etiology of psoriatic arthritis is unknown, but is generally felt to be a spontaneous result of genetic and immunologic factors. Many similar immunologic cellular and cytokine pathways are activated in the skin and joint, promoting migration of immune cells to the site of inflammation and upregulating cellular activation at this site. As in psoriasis, there has been speculation regarding the possibility of infectious antigenic triggering in some cases of psoriatic arthritis.

Treatment

The treatment of psoriatic arthritis has been revolutionized by the recent development and use of new biological therapies, especially anti-TNF medications, for patients with moderate-to-severe disease. These agents have yielded significant advances in the effective treatment of symptoms and signs of both arthritis and enthesitis. Furthermore, new evidence of inhibition or slowing of radiological signs of disease progression suggests that that these drugs may have the potential to alter the natural history of psoriatic arthritis.

Indications for systemic therapy. While aggressive disease warrants aggressive therapy with biological agents to prevent premature morbidity and possibly early mortality, patients who have stable milder disease will not need such treatment. It is therefore important to determine an appropriate therapeutic strategy that takes into account patient and disease characteristics.

It is appropriate to use systemic disease-modifying therapies when one or more of the following pertain:

- there is active disease (i.e. persistent inflammation in several joints despite efforts at control with NSAIDs)
- the patient is unable to pursue activities of daily living, work or recreation relatively easily
- the ESR and/or CRP levels are elevated
- many joints are involved
- there is radiographic evidence of erosions.

By contrast, patients with milder disease manifestations may be adequately controlled with NSAID therapy. The recently introduced cyclo-oxygenase 2 (COX-2) inhibitors, while not offering superior efficacy, do offer better gastrointestinal tolerance and safety. Long-term therapy with COX-2 inhibitors is therefore quite feasible in patients with mild disease. If a patient has just one or two joints that are actively inflamed, or a joint disproportionately inflamed in comparison with others, then selective corticosteroid injection can be helpful (Table 9.3).

Drug therapy is bolstered by physical and occupational therapy and exercise to maintain strength in the muscles around inflamed joints and to help prevent joint damage.

Traditional agents. The traditional pattern of medication use for systemic therapy of psoriatic arthritis has been largely derived from our experience in treating rheumatoid arthritis. Methotrexate, sulfasalazine, ciclosporin and a newer agent, leflunomide, are used. Hydroxychloroquine and corticosteroids are also prescribed, but less commonly than the aforementioned agents because of their tendency to aggravate skin disease.

Methotrexate is widely used for psoriatic arthritis despite the fact that the only controlled trial showed marginal results (with doses of 7.5 mg and 15 mg) in both the joint and skin. Current dosage regimens are 15–25 mg/week, with monitoring of complete blood count and liver function tests every 8 weeks. These doses can yield clinically meaningful improvements in both joint and skin disease. Guidelines for methotrexate use in psoriasis, including

TABLE 9.3

Therapies for psoriatic arthritis

Mild arthritis symptoms
- Non-steroidal anti-inflammatory drugs
- Physiotherapy
- Occupational therapy
- Exercise
- Selective local corticosteroid injection

Moderate-to-severe arthritis symptoms

Use same approaches as for mild disease plus:
- Non-biological therapies:
  - methotrexate
  - sulfasalazine
  - leflunomide
  - ciclosporin
  - azathioprine
- Biological therapies:
  - approved: etanercept
  - in development: infliximab, adalimumab, alefacept, anakinra
- Combination of non-biological and biological therapies

periodic liver biopsy, are discussed in Chapter 6. Concomitant use of folic acid, 1 mg/day, reduces the risk of mouth ulcers as well as other risks associated with impaired liver function.

Symptomatic side effects include nausea and, rarely, diarrhea and hair loss. An extremely rare side effect is acute interstitial lung disease. Hepatotoxicity remains the major concern with long-term use.

Sulfasalazine, 2 g/day, has been shown to be beneficial, albeit marginally, for joint disease, but has not been shown to improve skin lesions. Side effects are minimal and include rare gastrointestinal discomfort and diarrhea.

Ciclosporin has shown rapid and significant effects on skin lesions but, unfortunately, yields only marginal improvement in the joints. Furthermore, side effects of hypertension and renal insufficiency limit its dosing and duration of use.

Leflunomide, a pyrimidine inhibitor, has recently been shown in a controlled trial to improve joint and skin inflammation when used in a standard dose of 20 mg/day. This drug has a similar side effect profile to methotrexate, so monitoring for blood count and liver function test abnormalities is mandated.

Hydroxychloroquine, an antimalarial commonly used to treat mild rheumatoid arthritis, is useful in milder cases of psoriatic arthritis. However, its use has been curtailed partly because of the rare risk of flaring of psoriasis. Side effects with this drug are usually minimal. Periodic ophthalmological examination is suggested because of the extremely minor potential for retinopathy.

Systemic corticosteroids must be used judiciously, because patients may experience a post-steroid flaring of psoriasis on withdrawal. There is also a risk of osteopenia or osteoporosis with chronic use.

Biological response modifiers. The advent of biological therapy, particularly anti-TNF agents, has provided a major breakthrough in the management of psoriatic arthritis (see Chapter 8). Well controlled trials of two anti-TNF medications have been conducted, in which etanercept was given in a standard dose of 25 mg subcutaneously twice a week and infliximab was administered in a standard induction regimen of three infusions of 5 mg/kg over 6 weeks followed by maintenance therapy every 2 months. Dramatic improvements were noted in all parameters of disease activity in the joints and skin, as well as significant improvements in quality of life measures. These agents work quickly as well as effectively for the majority of patients.

Etanercept is the first biologic to be approved for psoriatic arthritis. Long-term use (up to a year) has demonstrated that etanercept has sustained efficacy, as well as achieving significant halting or slowing of disease progression, as indicated by lack of radiological signs of deterioration. Other biological agents in development include infliximab, adalimumab, onercept, alefacept and anakinra.

As discussed in Chapter 8, the overall risk profile for the biologics appears to be superior to that of the traditional disease-modifying drugs. Hence, when the overall benefit is compared with the low risk potential, these agents represent a significant advance in the treatment of moderate-to-severe psoriatic arthritis.

Numerous other biological agents are likely to demonstrate efficacy in treating the musculoskeletal symptoms of psoriatic arthritis. Another anti-TNF medication, adalimumab, administered subcutaneously twice weekly, has been approved for treatment of rheumatoid arthritis, and is currently undergoing investigation in psoriatic arthritis and psoriasis. Other anti-TNF medications may follow.

T-cell regulatory medications, including alefacept and efalizumab, which have already been approved or are expected to receive approval soon for the treatment of psoriasis, are being tested for efficacy in psoriatic arthritis, with efaluzimab recently found to be marginally superior to placebo. A number of new compounds with novel biological targets are currently being tested in rheumatoid arthritis or psoriasis and are likely also to be tested in psoriatic arthritis.

Rheumatology–dermatology teamwork

Given the overlapping capability of drugs to treat both the skin and the joint manifestations of psoriatic arthritis, it is advantageous for the primary care physician, dermatologist and rheumatologist to work together to manage both skin and joints optimally and to synchronize therapeutic approaches. Many patients with psoriatic arthritis are managed primarily by a dermatologist – or in some situations by their primary care physician – for the skin manifestations of their disease. Hence, there is a unique opportunity for these physicians to recognize joint disease and potentially initiate treatment. At the very least, it is imperative that all involved physicians remain alert to the possibility of joint disease since, in a proportion of patients, progressive joint destruction will occur in the absence of effective therapy. This progression may now be ameliorated or prevented with the use of the newer anti-TNFα agents, with etanercept approved in the USA for the treatment of psoriatic arthritis.

It can be important to involve a rheumatologist early to confirm the diagnosis of psoriatic arthritis, to help formulate appropriate therapeutic strategies, to work with difficult-to-treat cases, and to triage care to other members of the management team, such as physiotherapists and orthopedics specialists.

Key points – psoriatic arthritis

- Psoriatic arthritis is often underdiagnosed and undertreated; however, it is important to recognize this disease because advances in therapy offer the prospect of more complete disease control.
- The most common initial variant of psoriatic arthritis is oligoarticular, asymmetrical arthritis, but with time the disease becomes more polyarticular and symmetrical.
- The traditional approach to systemic therapy for psoriatic arthritis has relied on the experience derived from treatment of rheumatoid arthritis.
- The anti-TNF medication etanercept is effective in the treatment of the signs and symptoms of moderate-to-severe psoriatic arthritis.
- Infliximab and adalimumab are currently under investigation for similar properties.
- There is evidence to suggest that anti-TNF agents can slow radiographic disease progression.
- Optimal management requires a team approach.

Key references

Gladman DD. Psoriatic arthritis. In: Maddison PJ, Isenberg DA, Glass DN, eds. *Oxford Textbook of Rheumatology.* Oxford: Oxford University Press, 1998; 1071–84.

Gladman DD, Brockbank J. Psoriatic arthritis. *Expert Opin Investig Drugs* 2000;9:1511–22.

Jones G, Crotty M, Brooks P. Interventions for treating psoriatic arthritis (Cochrane Review). Oxford: The Cochrane Library, 2001.

Mease PJ. Current treatment of psoriatic arthritis. *Rheum Dis Clin North Am* 2003;29:495–511.

Mease PJ. Psoriatic arthritis/psoriasis. In: Smolen JS, Lipsky PE, eds. *Targeted Therapies in Rheumatology.* New York: Martin Dunitz, 2003;525–48.

There has been significant progress in our scientific understanding of the causes and mechanisms underlying psoriasis. This improved insight into the disease, together with the advent of more specific targeted therapies, will alter the way in which the disease is managed in the future.

Pathogenesis

Identification of the genes responsible for psoriasis is likely to have far-reaching implications for future clinical practice. Elucidation of the genetic profile of an individual might allow the physician to give an accurate prognosis, particularly relating to future development of psoriatic arthritis (skin signs usually precede joint signs by 5–10 years). Genetic profiling might also allow the response to particular therapies to be predicted, thus rationalizing drug prescribing.

Already, gene chip technology has allowed the identification of several genetic markers for psoriasis. One recent study was able to separate psoriatic patients from normal controls solely on the basis of gene expression.

Further spin-offs of genetic research may include the identification of environmental triggers for psoriasis.

Discovery of disease-specific biological pathways may lead to new models for drug discovery, more specific treatments and the development of diagnostic and prognostic aids. The various clinical forms of psoriasis are generally easy to diagnose, but in the few cases in which there is doubt, diagnostic testing would be of enormous benefit.

Systemic medications

Our understanding of the immunologic basis for psoriasis has led to the development of a range of novel, highly specific immunotherapeutic biological compounds for the treatment of moderate-to-severe disease.

Antisense technology. Preclinical and clinical trials are in progress to evaluate medications that take into account the genes implicated in psoriasis. Antisense technology allows the blockade of specific genes, which results in reduced gene expression.

ISIS-104838 is an antisense oligonucleotide specific for TNFα messenger RNA (mRNA). By binding to the mRNA, the antisense agent inhibits the synthesis of TNFα. This medication, which is given either intravenously or subcutaneously, is in phase II trials, as is a topical formulation.

Preclinical evaluation of an anti-insulin-like growth factor (anti-IGF) antisense oligonucleotide is also under way. IGF-I receptor (IGF-IR) regulates keratinocyte mitogenic and antiapoptotic signaling. Fogarty and colleagues produced sequence-specific antisense inhibition of IGF-IR in a human keratinocyte line.

Biological response modifiers. More than 15 biological response modifiers are in various stages of clinical trials. These medications have the potential to induce longer remissions with less toxicity than our current armamentarium (see Chapter 8).

Future trends in the biologics field include focusing on other aspects of the immune system and targeting more specific immune aberrances involved in the pathogenesis of psoriasis.

The optimal ways of combining biological therapies with traditional therapies such as phototherapy, retinoids, methotrexate and topical treatments should become apparent as the results of current studies become available. Eventually, it may be possible to add multiple biological therapies into a combination or sequential regimen.

Retinoids. Another systemic drug worthy of mention is an oral formulation of tazarotene. (The topical form of this receptor-selective retinoid is already available for the treatment of plaque psoriasis.) The results of a recent phase III trial for oral tazarotene show it to be at least as effective as acitretin but without some of the more serious side effects (such as alopecia, abnormal liver function tests and abnormal cholesterol/triglycerides).

Oral pimecrolimus. The topical form of this calcineurin inhibitor has been used for several years, but an oral preparation is not yet commercially available. Recent data from researchers at the University of Vienna, Austria, demonstrate a marked improvement in psoriasis symptoms with oral pimecrolimus over a 12-week study period. Phase III studies will attempt to answer questions regarding ideal dosing and the side effect profile.

Peptide T is a chain of eight amino acids that mimics a portion of the outer envelope protein, gp120, of HIV-1. It appears to be involved with the attachment of HIV-1 to helper T cells. Peptide T is given as an intravenous infusion and has demonstrated both anti-inflammatory and antichemotactic properties. Raychaudhuri speculates that this agent is beneficial in psoriasis by causing a shift in cytokine profile from TH-1 to TH-2. Small studies have demonstrated promising results.

Topical medications
Since publication of the previous edition of *Fast Facts – Psoriasis*, several new topical medications have been approved for use in psoriasis, and others are being evaluated.

Calcineurin inhibitors prevent transcription of proinflammatory cytokines that mediate psoriasis and other inflammatory dermatoses. Two agents, tacrolimus and pimecrolimus, are available in topical formulation. Tacrolimus is a macrolide and pimecrolimus is an ascomycin derivative; both have significant anti-inflammatory effects. These two medications are approved by the US Food and Drug Administration for the treatment of eczema, but do not appear to work well for standard psoriasis plaques. However, they appear helpful for psoriasis on the face and intertriginous areas and, unlike topical steroids, do not produce striae and telangiectasia.

Topical ciclosporin has poor skin penetration because of its molecular size and lipophilicity. Various formulations that may increase the topical availability of this agent are being evaluated.

Photodynamic therapy

Two new photodynamic agents, MV9411 and verteporfin, are currently in phase II trials.

MV9411, a topical gel medication, acts as a skin photosensitizing agent, augmenting the effects of light therapy for the treatment of plaque psoriasis. Only those areas specifically treated with the topical medication are affected. This effect therefore reduces the general light exposure.

Verteporfin is an intravenous photosensitizing agent used with UV light.

Changes in clinical practice

The increasing cost of healthcare delivery has resulted in a worldwide reduction in the number of inpatient beds available for dermatology patients. This means that patients with psoriasis are less likely to receive traditional treatments such as Ingram's regimen (dithranol and UVB phototherapy) in hospital. As a consequence, day-care centers have been established, staffed by dermatologically trained nurses capable of delivering complex topical treatment and phototherapy. Such facilities are expanding rapidly. This change in clinical practice has also led to an increase in the use of community-based care and nurse practitioners for patients with psoriasis.

Increasingly, physicians and investigators are using psychosocial instruments to monitor the effectiveness of therapy and techniques that complement established therapies. The aim of employing such instruments is to reduce the potentially serious impact that psoriasis and its treatments have on patients' quality of life.

The recognition that psoriasis has a significant impact on the quality of life of all affected individuals (physically and emotionally), as well as the realization that psoriatic arthritis is as common as rheumatoid arthritis, will intensify the need for more systemic therapies to be made available.

All these changes are to be welcomed, and the outlook for patients with psoriasis, provided that appropriate healthcare resources are available, is now much brighter.

Key references

Bowcock AM, Shannon W, Du F et al. Insights into psoriasis and other inflammatory diseases from large-scale gene expression studies. *Hum Mol Genet* 2001;10: 1793–1805.

Farber EM, Cohen EN, Trozak DJ, Wilkinson DI. Peptide T improves psoriasis when infused into lesions in nanogram amounts. *J Am Acad Dermatol* 1991;25:658–64.

Fogarty RD, McKean SC, White PJ et al. Sequence dependence of C5-propynyl-dU,dC-phosphoro-thioate oligonucleotide inhibition of the human IGF-I receptor: mRNA, protein, and cell growth. *Antisense Nucleic Acid Drug Dev* 2002;12:369–77.

Freeman AK, Linowski GJ, Brady C et al. Tacrolimus ointment for the treatment of psoriasis on the face and intertriginous areas. *J Am Acad Dermatol* 2003;48: 564–8.

Kennewell P. Technology evaluation: ISIS-104838, OraSense. *Curr Opin Mol Ther* 2003;5: 76–80.

Koo J. Result of phase III trials of an oral gel-capsule formulation of tazarotene in the treatment of moderate to severe psoriasis. American Academy of Dermatology 61st annual meeting. 21–26 March 2003, San Francisco, California.

Marcusson JA, Talme T, Wetterberg L, Johansson O. Peptide T a new treatment for psoriasis? A study of nine patients. *Acta Derm Venereol* 1991;71: 479–83.

Raychaudhuri SP, Farber EM, Raychaudhuri SK. Immuno-modulatory effects of peptide T on Th 1/Th 2 cytokines. *Int J Immunopharmacol* 1999;21: 609–15.

Raychaudhuri SK, Raychaudhuri SP, Farber EM. Anti-chemotactic activities of peptide-T: a possible mechanism of actions for its therapeutic effects on psoriasis. *Int J Immunopharmacol* 1998;20: 661–7.

Useful addresses

USA

National Psoriasis Foundation
6600 SW 92nd Avenue
Suite 300
Portland, OR 97223-7195
Tel: +1 503 244 7404
Fax: +1 503 245 0626
www.psoriasis.org

UK

The Psoriasis Association
7 Milton Street
Northampton NN2 7JG
Tel: +44 (0)1604 711 129
Fax: +44 (0)1604 792 894
mail@psoriasis.demon.co.uk
www.psoriasis-
association.org.uk

**The Alliance for Action on
Psoriasis and Psoriatic Arthritis**
PO Box 111
St Albans, Herts AL2 3JQ
Tel: 0870 770 3212
Fax: 0870 770 3213
info@paalliance.org
www.paalliance.org

International

**International Federation of
Psoriasis Associations (IFPA)**
6600 SW 92nd Avenue
Suite 300
Portland, OR 97223-7195
USA
Tel: +1 503 244 7404
Fax: +1 503 245 0626
getinfo@ifpa-pso.org
www.ifpa-pso.org
The IFPA's membership comprises
lay psoriasis organizations from
many countries around the world.
IFPA members meet regularly to
collaborate and to discuss issues
affecting people with psoriasis.

Australia

The Psoriasis Association
16 Musgrave Street
Kirra, Qld 4225
Tel: +61 (0)7 5599 1166
Fax: +61 (0)7 5599 1166
info@psoriasis.org.au
www.psoriasis.org.au

New Zealand

Psoriasis Association of New Zealand
PO Box 44007
Lower Hutt, Wellington 6315
Tel: +64 (0)4 568 7139
Fax: +64 (0)4 568 7149
psoriasis@xtra.co.nz
www.everybody.co.nz/support/
psoriasis.html

Canada

Psoriasis Society of Canada
PO Box 25015
Halifax, Nova Scotia, B3M 4H4
Tel: +1 902 443 8680
Toll-free: 800 656 4494
Fax: +1 902 443 2073
www.psoriasissociety.org

Singapore

Psoriasis Association of Singapore
c/o National Skin Centre
No. 1 Mandalay Road
Singapore 308205
Tel: +65 6350 8551
Fax: +65 6253 3225
psoriasis@association.org.sg

South Africa

South African Psoriasis Association
PO Box 801
Brackenfell, Cape 7561
Tel/fax: +27 21 981 1650
cathalex@sybaweb.co.za

Index